Cardiology Board Review

Cardiology Board Review

ECG, Hemodynamic and Angiographic Unknowns

Edited by

George A. Stouffer, MD
University of North Carolina
Chapel Hill, NC
USA

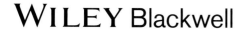

Registered Office(s)
John Wiley & Sons, Inc., 111 River Street, Hoboken, NJ 07030, USA
John Wiley & Sons Ltd, The Atrium, Southern Gate, Chichester, West Sussex, PO19 8SQ, UK

Editorial Office
9600 Garsington Road, Oxford, OX4 2DQ, UK

For details of our global editorial offices, customer services, and more information about Wiley products visit us at www.wiley.com.

Wiley also publishes its books in a variety of electronic formats and by print-on-demand. Some content that appears in standard print versions of this book may not be available in other formats.

Library of Congress Cataloging-in-Publication Data

Names: Stouffer, George A., editor.
Title: Cardiology board review : ECG, hemodynamic, and angiographic unknowns / edited by George A. Stouffer.
Description: Hoboken, NJ : Wiley-Blackwell, 2019. | Includes bibliographical references and index. |
Identifiers: LCCN 2019003180 (print) | LCCN 2019004188 (ebook) | ISBN 9781119423256 (Adobe PDF) | ISBN 9781119423249 (ePub) | ISBN 9781119423232 (pbk.)
Subjects: | MESH: Heart Diseases–diagnosis | Electrocardiography | Hemodynamics | Examination Question | Case Reports
Classification: LCC RC683.5.E5 (ebook) | LCC RC683.5.E5 (print) | NLM WG 18.2 | DDC 616.1/207547–dc23
LC record available at https://lccn.loc.gov/2019003180

Cover Design: Wiley
Cover Images: © ronstik/Shutterstock, © George A. Stouffer

Set in 10/12pt Warnock by SPi Global, Pondicherry, India
Printed and bound in Singapore by Markono Print Media Pte Ltd

10 9 8 7 6 5 4 3 2 1

This book is dedicated to my wife Meg and my four children (Mark, Jeanie, Joy, and Anna) for all the joy they bring into my life.

Contents

Cases compiled with contributions from

Amir Aghajanian MD
University of North Carolina
Chapel Hill, NC, USA

Destiny Davis BS
University of North Carolina
Chapel Hill, NC, USA

Allie Goins MD
Emory University
Atlanta, GA, USA

David Lee MD
University of North Carolina
Chapel Hill, NC, USA

Shiv Madan MD
University of North Carolina
Chapel Hill, NC, USA

Greg Means MD
University of North Carolina
Chapel Hill, NC, USA

Ryan Orgel MD
University of North Carolina
Chapel Hill, NC, USA

Anand Shah BS
Duke University
Durham, NC, USA

Craig Sweeney BS
University of North Carolina
Chapel Hill, NC, USA

Cynthia Zhou BS
University of North Carolina
Chapel Hill, NC, USA

Preface

This book provides a general overview of the basics of cardiology presented in a case-based format. I have found in my career that information presented in the form of specific cases can supplement information presented in standard textbook format as it enables a discussion of multiple factors which influence the diagnosis and management of a specific patient and also enhances retention of the material. This book revolves around many interesting patients, with each of the cases being drawn from real life. As this book illustrates, each patient has something to teach us.

This book covers a wide spectrum of cases including congenital heart disease, coronary artery disease, cardiomyopathies, valvular heart disease, arrhythmias, heart failure, peripheral vascular disease, cerebral vascular disease, congenital heart disease, and pericardial disease. It is designed to be a valuable resource to the cardiologist or cardiologist in training and to provide an understanding of pathophysiology, diagnostic methods, and treatment of patients with cardiovascular disease.

Cardiology Board Review is also designed to be used for review for the Cardiovascular Disease Certification Examination and other cardiology examinations. This book will supplement more standard Board review books by discussing guideline recommendations in a case review format.

This book includes numerous images such as electrocardiograms, angiograms, and pressure tracings. Image interpretation is one of the most fundamental and valuable clinical skills for the clinical cardiologist, but "how-to" books run the risk of losing the user in a series of tracings that are not presented in a clinical framework and thus are boring to read and difficult to remember. In this book, images are presented in the context of a patient with a specific complaint. Rather than an exhaustive discussion of imaging, this book focuses on ECGs, angiograms, and pressure tracings provide important information in the diagnosis of specific cardiovascular disease states.

Case 1: A 31-Year-Old Man with Fever and Rapidly Progressive Dyspnea

A 31-year-old man with a history of ankylosing spondylitis is brought to the Emergency Department by a friend. He reports one week of low-grade fevers (100.5 °F), cough, progressive shortness of breath, nausea, diarrhea, and occasional vomiting. He has noticed a rapid decline in his exercise tolerance in the past week and states he can't even walk more than 10–20 ft without getting very short of breath. The patient also complains of a frothy cough sometimes laced with blood, paroxysmal nocturnal dyspnea, and orthopnea. He denies any chest pain.

On physical examination, blood pressure is 110/40 mmHg, pulse rate is 110 bpm, and oxygen saturation is 98%. His lungs are clear and he has a diastolic murmur along the right upper sternal border. After an echocardiogram, he is referred for cardiac catheterization. What is the diagnosis based on the aortogram below (Figure 1.1)?

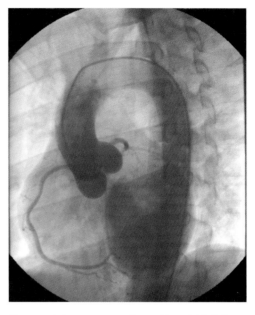

Figure 1.1 Aortogram performed in an LAO (left anterior oblique) projection. The pigtail catheter is located right above the aortic valve during injection of contrast dye.

Aortic Regurgitation

The pigtail catheter is in the aortic root and a power injection of a high volume of contrast is performed. This results in filling of the left ventricle, consistent with aortic regurgitation (AR). Angiographic classification of severity of AR is based on the amount of contrast dye entering the left ventricle during an aortogram:

- 1+ some dye enters ventricle but clears with every systole
- 2+ the ventricle becomes completely opacified after several heartbeats and remains opacified throughout the cardiac cycle
- 3+ after several heartbeats – the ventricle becomes as dark as the aorta
- 4+ after several heartbeats – the ventricle becomes darker than the aorta

Cardiology Board Review: ECG, Hemodynamic and Angiographic Unknowns, First Edition. Edited by George A. Stouffer.
© 2019 John Wiley & Sons Ltd. Published 2019 by John Wiley & Sons Ltd.

Note that in the 2014 AHA/ACC Valvular Heart Disease Guideline, transthoracic echocardiography is the first line diagnostic modality for AR as it provides information on the cause of regurgitation, regurgitant severity, and LV (left ventricular) size and systolic function. Cardiac magnetic resonance imaging is indicated in patients with AR in whom echocardiographic images are suboptimal. Cardiac catheterization was performed in this patient to evaluate coronary anatomy prior to surgery.

AR is a condition of increased afterload with associated hemodynamic changes varying depending on the time–course of the valve dysfunction. If AR develops rapidly (i.e. acute or subacute AR), the left ventricle is unable to handle the pressure and volume overload causing a rapid increase in left ventricular pressures during diastole, markedly elevated pressures at end diastole, and premature closure of the mitral valve. Systemic diastolic pressures may be low but generally there is a minimal increase in pulse pressure; in very severe cases of acute AR, cardiac output may fall leading to a decrease in pulse pressure and/or hypotension. In chronic AR, stroke volume increases to maintain effective forward flow. This leads to dilation of the left ventricle, leading in some patients to the development of a massively dilated left ventricle, termed *cor bovinum*.

In this patient, an echocardiogram showed severely decreased left ventricular contraction with left atrial dilation. The aortic valve was trileaflet with inadequate coaptation and severe AR (Table 1.1). Right ventricular contractile performance was decreased. Hemodynamic changes of severe AR were found at cardiac catheterization including elevated left ventricular end diastolic pressure (38 mmHg), equalization of aortic and left ventricular pressures during diastole (Figure 1.2), and premature closure of the mitral valve during diastole. There was moderate pulmonary hypertension (50/33 mmHg) and reduced cardiac output (2.3 l/min by assumed Fick Method). The patient underwent successful aortic valve replacement with a 25 mm St. Jude prosthesis.

Ankylosing spondylitis is an autoimmune spondylarthropathy that is characterized by chronic, painful, degenerative inflammatory arthritis primarily affecting the lower spine and sacroiliac joints. There is a strong association with the class I major histocompatibility complex antigen HLA-B27. In patients with ankylosing spondylitis the incidence of AR is approximately 10%.

The 4 stages of AR according to the 2014 AHA/ACC Valvular Heart Disease Guideline are: Stage A: No current AR but at risk of developing AR (including bicuspid aortic valve, aortic valve sclerosis, diseases of the aortic sinuses or ascending aorta, history of

Table 1.1 Echo criteria for grading severity of aortic regurgitation (AR).

Echo criteria	Mild AR	Moderate AR	Severe AR
Doppler jet width	≤25% of LVOT	25–64% of LVOT	≥65% of LVOT
Vena Contracta	<0.3 cm	0.3–0.6 cm	>0.6 cm
Regurgitant volume	≤30 ml/beat	30–59 ml/beat	≥60 ml/beat
Regurgitant fraction	≤30%	30–49%	≥50%
Effective regurgitant orifice (ERO)	<0.1 cm^2	0.1–0.29 cm^2	≥0.3 cm^2
Miscellaneous			Holodiastolic flow reversal in the proximal abdominal aorta

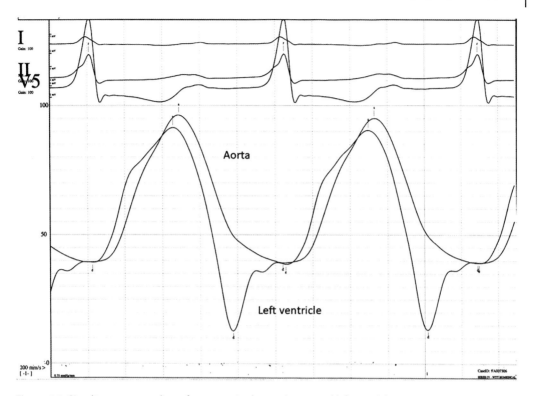

Figure 1.2 Simultaneous recording of pressures in the aortic root and left ventricle.

rheumatic fever or known rheumatic heart disease, infective endocarditis); Stage B: progressive mild-to-moderate AR; Stage C: severe asymptomatic; and Stage D: symptomatic AR.

Class 1 indications for aortic valve replacement in AR include: (i) Symptomatic patients with severe AR regardless of systolic function; (ii) Asymptomatic patients with chronic severe AR and LV systolic dysfunction (LVEF 50 mm or indexed LV end-systolic dimension [LVESD] >25 mm/m^2); and (iii) Patients undergoing cardiac surgery for other indications with severe AR (stage C or D). Class 2a indications include: (i) Asymptomatic patients with severe AR with normal LV systolic function (LVEF ≥50%) but with severe LV dilation (LVESD >50 mm or indexed LVESD >25 mm/m^2) and (ii) moderate AR (stage B) while undergoing surgery on the ascending aorta, coronary artery bypass grafting (CABG), or mitral valve surgery. Class 2b indication includes Asymptomatic patients with severe AR, normal LV systolic function at rest (LVEF ≥50%, stage C1), but with progressive severe LV dilatation (LV end-diastolic dimension >65 mm) if surgical risk is low.

Further Reading

Edhouse, J., Thakur, R.K., and Khalil, J.M. (2002). Clinical review: ABC of clinical electrocardiography: Conditions affecting the left side of the heart. *BMJ* 324: 1264–1267.

Goldbarg, S.H. and Halperin, J.L. (2008). Aortic regurgitation: disease progression and management. *Nature Clinical Practice. Cardiovascular Medicine* 5: 269–279.

Nishimura, R.A., Otto, C.M., Bonow, R.O. et al. (2014). 2014 AHA/ACC guideline for the management of patients with valvular heart disease: a report of the American

College of Cardiology/American Heart Association Task Force on Practice Guidelines. *Journal of the American College of Cardiology* 63 (22): e57–e185.

Rigby, W.F.C., Fan, C.-M., and Mark, E.J. (2002). Case 39-2002 – A 35-year-old man with headache, deviation of the tongue, and unusual radiographic abnormalities. *The New England Journal of Medicine* 347: 2057–2065.

Stouffer, G.A. (ed.) (2017). *Aortic regurgitation in Cardiovascular Hemodynamics for the Clinician*, 2e. Blackwell Publishing.

Case 2: A Young Man with Palpitations After a Party

You are asked to see a 26-year-old man who presented to the Emergency Department at 1 a.m. complaining of sudden onset of a rapid heartbeat. He was "celebrating" (it is not clear what) earlier this evening and has consumed a large quantity of alcohol. He has no significant past medical history and no family history of premature sudden death. What does the ECG show (Figure 2.1)?

Atrial Fibrillation

The ECG shows an irregular, narrow complex tachycardia at a rate of approximately 150 bpm. The lack of P waves and presence of oscillatory f waves (small, irregular waves seen as a rapid-cycle baseline fluctuation) point to atrial fibrillation. The various amplitudes of QRS complexes and variable RR intervals are also

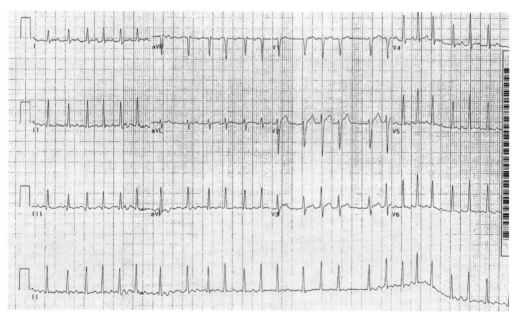

Figure 2.1 ECG on presentation.

Cardiology Board Review: ECG, Hemodynamic and Angiographic Unknowns, First Edition. Edited by George A. Stouffer.
© 2019 John Wiley & Sons Ltd. Published 2019 by John Wiley & Sons Ltd.

consistent with atrial fibrillation. Atrial fibrillation is a disorganized and nonsynchronous series of fibrillatory waves at a rate of 400–700 bpm that, in the majority of cases, originate within the pulmonary veins (recognition of this fact has led to the development of pulmonary vein isolation as a form of atrial fibrillation ablation). Atrioventricular (AV) node conduction is variable leading to the irregularly irregular rhythm which is typical of atrial fibrillation. The ventricular response to atrial fibrillation depends on many factors, but is determined by the number of impulses that overcome the AV node's refractory period and the His-Purkinje system's refractory period to reach the ventricles.

There are two arrhythmias which cause the vast majority of irregular, narrow complex tachycardias: atrial fibrillation and multifocal atrial tachycardia (MAT), with atrial fibrillation being the most common arrhythmia in clinical practice while MAT is rare. MAT occurs when there are various sites within the atria which have increased automaticity and thus compete to serve as controlling pacemakers. This rhythm is distinguished by the presence of P waves with at least three distinct morphologies (Figure 2.2). MAT is generally seen in older adults and usually occurs in the presence of significant comorbidity such as advanced lung disease or congestive heart failure. Wandering atrial pacemaker is the name of the rhythm when there are three or more P wave morphologies and the rate is less than 100 bpm.

Atrial fibrillation can be classified as: (i) recent onset (<48 hours); (ii) paroxysmal (terminates within seven days); (iii) persistent (>1 week but potentially subject to cardioversion); (iv) long-standing persistent (continuous atrial fibrillation for >12 months); or (v) permanent (patient and physician decide to not pursue any further efforts at cardioversion). Recurrent atrial fibrillation occurs when a patient develops two or more episodes of the disorder, which could be paroxysmal or persistent in nature. Paroxysmal atrial fibrillation is diagnosed if the episodes stop spontaneously within seven days, but is regarded as persistent if electrical or pharmacological cardioversion is needed to stop the arrhythmia. Permanent atrial fibrillation occurs when the patient remains in the arrhythmia as cardioversion is either not successful or deemed inappropriate. Sustained atrial fibrillation causes changes in electrophysiology and structure properties of atrium (a process known as atrial remodeling) that makes the atrium more susceptible to the initiation and maintenance of atrial fibrillation (atrial fibrillation begets atrial fibrillation).

Atrial fibrillation is generally a disease of aging. The prevalence of atrial fibrillation is less than 0.5% in young adults but increases to approximately 10% in individuals older than 80 years. Generally accepted causes of atrial fibrillation in young adults include hyperthyroidism, valvular heart disease, cardiomyopathy, electrocution, acute myocardial infarction, acute pericarditis, acute myocarditis, acute pulmonary embolus, cardiac trauma, amyloidosis, and pheochromocytoma. Atrial fibrillation caused by vagal stimulation (e.g. vomiting) and familial atrial fibrillation have been described. Lone atrial fibrillation is defined by the presence of atrial fibrillation with a structurally normal heart and no evidence of other precipitating cause. Lastly, other potential causes such as sleep apnea, tall stature, and obesity have also been proposed. In this individual, excessive alcohol consumption was thought to trigger the arrhythmia.

Holiday Heart syndrome is defined as an acute cardiac rhythm and/or conduction disturbance, most commonly supraventricular tachyarrhythmia, associated with heavy alcohol consumption in a person without other

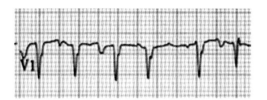

Figure 2.2 Rhythm strip showing different P wave morphologies that are found in wandering atrial pacemaker (rate <100 bpm) and multifocal atrial tachycardia (MAT) (rate ≥100 bpm).

clinical evidence of heart disease. Typically, this resolves rapidly with spontaneous recovery during subsequent abstinence from alcohol use. Atrial fibrillation is the most common arrhythmia observed with Holiday Heart syndrome but atrial flutter, junctional tachycardia, increased ectopics, and other arrhythmias have been reported. The etiology of the Holiday Heart syndrome is controversial but alcohol has been shown to possess direct proarrhythmic properties, especially in susceptible individuals.

Atrial fibrillation in young individuals due to excessive alcohol consumption is generally well-tolerated and self-limited. There are however case reports of sudden death. It is worth noting that in the presence of pre-excitation (an accessory pathway), atrial fibrillation can be a fatal arrhythmia. The lack of the normal rate control mechanism provided by the AV node can result in 1:1 transmission from the atria to the ventricles with resulting ventricular rates greater than 300 bpm (Figure 2.3).

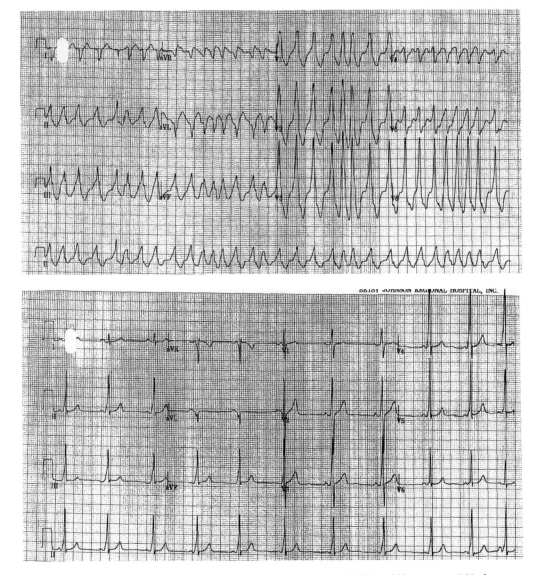

Figure 2.3 Atrial fibrillation in an individual with an accessory atrioventricular (AV) nodal bypass tract. ECG after cardioversion shows clear ECG evidence of Wolff-Parkinson-White Syndrome with a short PR interval and delta waves.

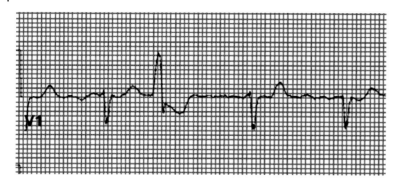

Figure 2.4 An example of Ashman's phenomenon.

The ACCF/AHA guidelines recommend the following evaluation in a patient with new onset atrial fibrillation: "An ECG, or other electrocardiographic recording, is the essential tool for confirming AF. A chest radiograph should be done if pulmonary disease or heart failure is suspected and may also detect enlargement of the cardiac chambers. As part of the initial evaluation, all patients with AF should have a 2-dimensional transthoracic echocardiogram to detect underlying structural heart disease, assess cardiac function, and evaluate atrial size. Additional laboratory evaluation should include assessment of serum electrolytes and of thyroid, renal, and hepatic function, and a blood count."

One special situation that can occur on the ECG of a patient with atrial fibrillation deserves mention. Ashman's phenomenon is an aberrantly conducted supraventricular beat that occurs in atrial fibrillation (Figure 2.4). This phenomenon is due to the relationship of cycle length and cardiac repolarization and can be recognized on a rhythm strip by noting a wide complex beat occurring after a short RR interval that follows immediately after a much longer RR interval. The mechanism of this phenomenon is due to the fact that the rate of repolarization of the cardiac conduction system is dependent upon heart rate. Repolarization is relatively slow when the heart rate is slow but increases as the heart rate increases. Right bundle branch block morphology is common in Ashman's phenomenon because the right bundle branch is slower to repolarize than the left bundle branch. Ashman's phenomenon generally occurs in patients with atrial fibrillation when the heart rate is relatively constant and well controlled.

Further Reading

January, C.T., Wann, L.S., Alpert, J.S. et al. (2014). 2014 AHA/ACC/HRS guideline for the management of patients with atrial fibrillation: a report of the American College of Cardiology/American Heart Association Task Force on Practice Guidelines and the Heart Rhythm Society. *Journal of the American College of Cardiology* 64 (21): e1–e76.

Kirchhof, P., Benussi, S., Kotecha, D. et al. (2016). 2016 ESC Guidelines for the management of atrial fibrillation developed in collaboration with EACTS. *European Heart Journal* 37 (38): 2893–2962.

Case 3: A 45-Year-Old Man with Chest Pain After an Automobile Accident

You are asked to see a 45-year-old man with no significant past medical history in the Emergency Department following a motor vehicle collision. He was slowing to a stop in a sedan when his car was hit from behind by a semi-trailer truck traveling 40 mi/h. He was wearing a seat belt and the airbag did not deploy. He denies any head trauma or loss of consciousness surrounding the event. He was able to get out of his car unassisted, and shortly thereafter developed constant, deep, substernal chest pain that he described as dull and 5 out of 10 in severity. He has no other associated symptoms such as shortness of breath, diaphoresis, nausea, or vomiting. The automated 12-lead electrocardiogram (ECG) interpretation is read as "ACUTE MI."

What is your interpretation of this ECG (Figure 3.1)?

Brugada Syndrome

This patient has Brugada pattern on his ECG which is described as a right bundle branch block (RBBB), normal QT internal, and persistent ST-segment elevation in leads V1 to V2-V3 that is not explainable by electrolyte

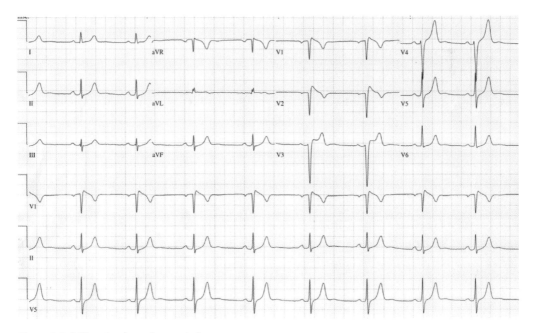

Figure 3.1 ECG at the time of presentation.

Cardiology Board Review: ECG, Hemodynamic and Angiographic Unknowns, First Edition. Edited by George A. Stouffer.
© 2019 John Wiley & Sons Ltd. Published 2019 by John Wiley & Sons Ltd.

derangements, ischemia, or structural heart disease (Brugada and Brugada 1992). According to the 2013 consensus statement on inherited arrhythmias, this pattern is definitively diagnosed when Brugada type 1 ST-segment elevation is observed either spontaneously or after administration of intravenous sodium channel-blocking agent in at least one precordial lead (V1 and V2) (Priori et al. 2013).

Clinical manifestations vary, and in the case of isolated Brugada pattern on ECG such as in this case, the patient may be asymptomatic. A patient who presents with the Brugada ECG criteria but without the clinical characteristics is said to have the Brugada pattern but not the syndrome. Diagnosis of Brugada Syndrome depends on both characteristic ECG findings (either spontaneous or inducible) and appropriate clinical findings (unexplained syncope, self-terminating polymorphic ventricular tachycardia, documented ventricular fibrillation, family history of sudden cardiac death at less than 45 years of age, Brugada ECG pattern in a family member, and/or inducibility of ventricular tachycardia by electrophysiologic study). The syndrome usually manifests during adulthood with a mean age of sudden death of 41 years. Other common symptoms include ventricular fibrillation or aborted sudden cardiac death, syncope, nocturnal agonal respiration, palpitations, or chest discomfort. These symptoms most frequently occur during rest or sleep, during a febrile state, or with vagotonic conditions. Rarely do symptoms manifest with exercise (Priori et al. 2013). The syndrome appears to be more common in persons of Asian descent (Alings and Wilde 1999), and men are 8–10 times more likely to be affected (Priori et al. 2013). These patients are at an increased risk of ventricular tachyarrhythmias and sudden cardiac death (Priori et al. 2013).

In this case, Brugada Syndrome was unrelated to the motor vehicle accident (the patient had no palpitations or loss of consciousness and the accident was not attributable to his error). Recognition of this pattern on ECG is very important however for at least two reasons: (i) interpretation of the ST elevation as an acute injury pattern would result in the faulty diagnosis of acute myocardial infarction or cardiac contusion; and (ii) individuals with Brugada Syndrome are at risk of sudden cardiac death and this patient should be further evaluated to see if he would benefit from primary prevention.

The Brugada Syndrome was initially described in 1992 by Brugada and Brugada who reported eight patients with a history of cardiac arrest and ECG findings of RBBB and ST-segment elevation in the right precordial leads and no evidence of any structural heart disease. Prior to that, the Centers for Disease Control and Prevention had reported cases of sudden death in young immigrants from Southeast Asia, described as Sudden Unexplained Death Syndrome (SUDS) which has subsequently been shown to be closely related to, if not the same as, the Brugada syndrome.

The Brugada Syndrome is an autosomal dominant genetic disorder with variable penetrance characterized by abnormal electrophysiologic activity in the right ventricular epicardium. Approximately one-fourth of cases are caused by loss of function mutations in the cardiac sodium channel SCN5A (abnormalities in this gene have also been linked to Long QT Syndrome 3). This gene encodes the α-subunit of the sodium ion channel and, when abnormal, results in increased inactivation of the sodium channel with a prolonged recovery time.

Three ECG patterns have been described in the Brugada Syndrome, with all three types having in common ST elevation ($\geq 2\,$mm at the J point) in the right precordial leads. In the "classic" Brugada ECG (type 1) the ST segment is continuously downsloping from the top of the R wave, is not elevated above baseline at the terminal portion and ends with an inverted T wave (such as in this patient). Types 2 and 3 have a "saddle-back" ST-T wave configuration (Figure 3.1). The ST segment descends toward the baseline with upward concavity and then rises again to an upright or biphasic

T wave. Type 2 is defined by the terminal portion of the ST segment being elevated ≤1 mm whereas in type 3 the terminal portion of the ST segment is elevated <1 mm. The ECG changes can be dynamic, with the same patient manifesting all three types at various points in time.

In some patients, complete or incomplete RBBB is present. In others, high take-off ST-segment elevation (accentuated J-point elevation) in the right precordial leads mimics the pattern of RBBB, but wide S waves in leads I, aVL, V_5, and V_6 typically seen in RBBB are absent (such as in this case). In these cases, the R in V1 is thought to be due to early repolarization of the right ventricular epicardium rather than a RBBB.

The Brugada pattern on ECG can be either persistent or inducible. Medications (including sodium channel blockers, cocaine, antidepressants, and antihistamines), electrolyte abnormalities, and acute illnesses may elicit ST-segment elevation in leads V_1 to V_3 in susceptible patients. To aide in the diagnosis, provocation testing by infusion of selected class IC antiarrhythmic drugs (e.g. flecainide or procainamide) can unmask the Brugada ECG pattern in affected subjects.

It is important to risk stratify patients based on clinical characteristics, as high-risk patients benefit from ICD (implantable cardioverter defibrillator) placement. The risk of lethal or near-lethal arrhythmic episodes among previously asymptomatic patients with Brugada pattern on ECG is estimated between 1 and 8% depending on the study. Irrespective of other predictors of outcome, patients with history of ventricular fibrillation are inherently high risk (Priori et al. 2013). Additionally, patients presenting with syncopal episodes in the presence of spontaneous Brugada type I ST elevation in leads V1–V2 have high rates of cardiac events in follow-up (Priori et al., 2002). These first two patient groups have a strong indication for ICD placement. Other indicators of increased risk are the presence of fragmented QRS, a refractory period of <200 ms, and male sex (Priori et al. 2013).

At this time, the only effective strategy for prevention of sudden cardiac death in patients with Brugada Syndrome is placement of an ICD. Please see Figure 3.2 for indications for ICD placement. Lifestyle modifications are also important for survival in Brugada Syndrome. There are numerous medications that may induce or aggravate ST-segment elevation in precordial leads, and patients with Brugada Syndrome are advised to avoid these. A complete list can be found at https://www.brugadadrugs.org. Additionally, all patients should avoid excessive alcohol intake, and immediately treat fevers with antipyretic drugs (Marquez et al. 2012).

Pharmacologic therapy focuses on inhibition of the transient outward potassium current or increasing the sodium and calcium currents. Isoproterenol increases the L-type calcium current and is useful in treatment of electrical storm in Brugada Syndrome (Priori et al. 2013). Quinidine is a class 1a antiarrhythmic drug that has been shown to prevent the induction of VF (ventricular fibrillation) and suppress spontaneous ventricular arrhythmias. Quinidine is used in patients with ICD who have been shocked multiple times, cases where ICD is contraindicated, and to suppress supraventricular arrhythmias (Marquez et al. 2012; Priori et al. 2013).

Catheter ablation of malignant arrhythmias is a promising future therapeutic avenue in Brugada Syndrome. Similar to pharmacologic treatment, there have been no randomized controlled trials addressing this issue, but Nademanee et al. (2011) completed a case series which showed that epicardial substrate ablation in the right ventricular outflow tract can prevent ventricular fibrillation inducibility in a high-risk population.

The patient was observed with serial ECGs, and cardiac troponin was collected every six hours and remained negative. His pain improved with anti-inflammatory medications and was thought to be due to musculoskeletal trauma rather than ischemia. He had high-risk findings on an electrophysiology study and an ICD was implanted.

Expert Consensus Recommendations on Brugada Syndrome Therapeutic Interventions	
Class I	1. The following lifestyle changes *are recommended* in all patients with diagnosis of BrS: a) Avoidance of drugs that may induce or aggravate ST-segment elevation in right precordial leads (for example, visit Brugadadrugs.org), b) Avoidance of excessive alcohol intake. c) Immediate treatment of fever with antipyretic drugs. 2. ICD implantation *is recommended* in patients with a diagnosis of BrS who: a) Are survivors of a cardiac arrest and/or b) Have documented spontaneous sustained VT with or without syncope.
Class IIa	3. ICD implantation *can be useful* in patients with a spontaneous diagnostic type I ECG who have a history of syncope judged to be likely caused by ventricular arrhythmias. 4. Quinidine *can be useful* in patients with a diagnosis of BrS and history of arrhythmic storms defined as more than two episodes of VT/VF in 24 hours. 5. Quinidine *can be useful* in patients with a diagnosis of BrS: a) Who qualify for an ICD but present a contraindication to the ICD or refuse it *and/or* b) Have a history of documented supraventricular arrhythmias that require treatment. 6. Isoproterenol infusion *can be useful* in suppressing arrhythmic storms in BrS patients.
Class IIb	7. ICD implantation *may be considered* in patients with a diagnosis of BrS who develop VF during programmed electrical stimulation (inducible patients). 8. Quinidine *may be considered* in asymptomatic patients with a diagnosis of BrS with a spontaneous **type I** ECG. 9. Catheter ablation *may be considered* in patients with a diagnosis of BrS and history of arrhythmic storms or repeated appropriate ICD shocks.
Class III	10. ICD implantation **is not indicated** in asymptomatic BrS patients with a drug-induced **type I** ECG and on the basis of a family history of SCD alone.

Figure 3.2 Consensus recommendations for ICD placement in patients with Brugada Syndrome. *Source:* Reproduced with the permission of Priori et al. (2013).

References

Alings, M. and Wilde, A. (1999). "Brugada" syndrome: clinical data and suggested pathophysiological mechanism. *Circulation* 99 (5): 666–673.

Brugada, P. and Brugada, J. (1992). Right bundle branch block, persistent ST segment elevation and sudden cardiac death: a distinct clinical and electrocardiographic syndrome. A multicenter report. *Journal of the American College of Cardiology* 20 (1396): 1391–1396.

Marquez, M.F., Bonny, A., Hernández-Castillo, E. et al. (2012). Long-term efficacy of low doses of quinidine on malignant arrhythmias in Brugada syndrome with an implantable cardioverter-defibrillator: a case series and literature review. *Heart Rhythm* 9 (12): 1995–2000.

Nademanee, K., Veerakul, G., Chandanamattha, P. et al. (2011). Prevention of ventricular fibrillation episodes in Brugada syndrome by catheter ablation over the anterior right ventricular outflow tract epicardium. *Circulation* 123 (12): 1270–1279.

Priori, S.G., Napolitano, C., Gasparini, M. et al. (2002). Natural history of Brugada syndrome: insights for risk stratification and management. *Circulation* 105 (11): 1342–1347.

Priori, S.G., Wilde, A.A., Horie, M. et al. (2013). HRS/EHRA/APHRS expert consensus statement on the diagnosis and management of patients with inherited primary arrhythmia syndromes: document endorsed by HRS, EHRA, and APHRS in May 2013 and by ACCF, AHA, PACES, and AEPC in June 2013. *Heart Rhythm* 10 (12): 1932–1963.

Case 4: A 67-Year-Old Man with Left-Sided Weakness

You are asked to see a 67-year-old man who presented to the Emergency Department with right homonymous hemianopia and left-sided weakness lasting four hours. He has known coronary artery disease (history of prior right coronary artery stent), hypertension, hyperlipidemia, diabetes, tonsillar squamous cell carcinoma of the neck treated with radiation therapy, and tobacco abuse. His current medical therapy includes beta-blocker, insulin, angiotensin converting enzyme inhibitor, and 81 mg daily of aspirin. Examination revealed a right-sided carotid bruit and no bruit on the left. He was diagnosed with a transient ischemia attack (TIA) and the Emergency Department physician wants your opinion on what diagnostic tests are needed.

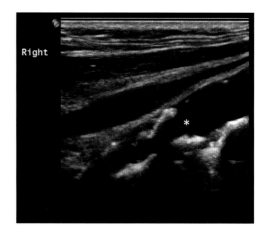

Figure 4.1 Carotid duplex study showing significant heterogeneous plaque with calcifications of the right internal carotid artery (ICA) (*: shows site of lesion).

Additional Evaluation

You recommend a carotid duplex examination which demonstrated a completely occluded left internal carotid artery (ICA), patent bilateral vertebral arteries, and a > 70% right ICA stenosis consisting of heterogeneous plaque with calcification (Figure 4.1). Clopidogrel 75 mg daily was started and aspirin was discontinued.

He underwent right carotid angiogram which revealed a calcified 80% stenosis (Figure 4.2a). Since he was deemed high risk for carotid endarterectomy (CEA) because of his previous neck radiation, this lesion was successfully treated with an 8 × 30 mm self-expanding carotid stent with 25% residual

stenosis (Figure 4.2b). A distal embolic protection device was used during the case which captured moderate debris. The patient tolerated the procedure without complication. Aspirin therapy in addition to clopidogrel was restarted for 30 days with the plan to be transitioned back to clopidogrel monotherapy. He also received continued therapy for secondary prevention of vascular disease including treatment with a statin and counseling on tobacco cessation.

Carotid Artery Disease

This case highlights a patient with sequelae of coronary artery and cerebrovascular disease likely driven by numerous underlying

Cardiology Board Review: ECG, Hemodynamic and Angiographic Unknowns, First Edition. Edited by George A. Stouffer.
© 2019 John Wiley & Sons Ltd. Published 2019 by John Wiley & Sons Ltd.

(a)   (b)

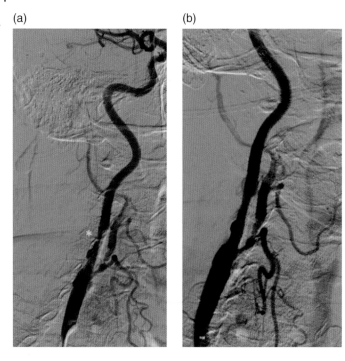

Figure 4.2 Right anterior oblique projection of right internal carotid angiogram revealing a calcified 80% stenosis pre- (A; *: shows site of lesion) and post-intervention (B).

risk factors including hyperlipidemia, diabetes, neck radiation, and tobacco abuse. Given findings of a significant right-sided internal carotid stenosis with an occluded left ICA in the setting of a TIA, revascularization was indicated to prevent a future, more severe cerebral vascular accident (CVA). Following his TIA which occurred while on aspirin monotherapy, his antiplatelet regimen was escalated to clopidogrel, a class 2b recommendation from the AHA/ASA 2006 guidelines based on the results of the Clopidogrel versus Aspirin in Patients at Risk of Ischaemic Events (CAPRIE) trial (CAPRIE Steering Committee 1996; Kernan et al. 2014).

Both CEA and carotid stenting were considered for revascularization but the previous neck radiation and contralateral carotid occlusion made surgical risk for CEA very high. Carotid stenting was successful and distal embolic protection was used to help reduce the risk of periprocedural stroke. Although there was not 100% luminal gain post-procedure, the aim of stenting is to cover the lesion to prevent further distal embolic events originating from the stenosis. In general, dual antiplatelet therapy after carotid stenting is recommended for at least 30 days with subsequent transition to monotherapy. Dual antiplatelet duration following carotid stenting is an important clinical question in need of more evidence.

Carotid Artery Disease – Clinical Presentation and Pathophysiology

Carotid artery disease is a narrowing of carotid artery lumen, usually by atherosclerotic plaque or calcification. Carotid disease has a large impact on public health as a common cause of ischemic CVA. Fifteen to twenty percent of ischemic strokes are thought to be caused by extracranial carotid disease (Wityk et al. 1996; Benjamin et al. 2010). Among survivors of stroke due to carotid disease, diagnosis and management is important as the risk for recurrent CVA can be as high as 25% by five years (Barnett et al. 1998). Carotid disease is an important mechanism for stroke via carotid dissection, acute thrombosis in the absence of contralateral blood supply or patent Circle of Willis, atheroembolism, and thromboembolism. Often, the presentation of TIA or CVA is manifested by stroke symptoms coming from the cerebral hemisphere supplied by the diseased artery of weakness, visual field defects, neglect, and/or aphasia. A common herald of carotid disease is amaurosis fugax, a painless and transient loss of vision due to retinal ischemia.

A carotid bruit may sometimes be auscultated on physical exam, but is an insensitive finding and may be absent in severe or totally occluded vessels. Although screening of totally asymptomatic individuals is not recommended, a bruit in a patient with risk factors or TIA/CVA should prompt consideration for non-invasive imaging (U.S. Preventive Services Task Force 2016). Options for imaging include carotid ultrasound, CT angiography (CTA), magnetic resonance angiography (MRA), and invasive catheter angiography. Consensus society guidelines recommend carotid ultrasound as a first-line imaging modality for patients with symptoms and high-risk asymptomatic patients (Brott et al. 2011).

Risk factor modification is the cornerstone of primary and secondary CVA prevention including treatment of hypertension, statin therapy of hyperlipidemia, and tobacco cessation. Antiplatelet options for secondary prevention of CVA include 75–325 mg aspirin, 75 mg clopidogrel, or the combination of aspirin plus dipyridamole. Due to increased bleeding events, secondary prevention of CVA with routine dual antiplatelet therapy with aspirin and clopidogrel or systemic anticoagulation with a vitamin K antagonist is not recommended (class 3 recommendation) (Brott et al. 2011). The exception to this is in the setting of presumed cardioembolic stroke (e.g. atrial fibrillation), where anticoagulation with a vitamin K antagonist or novel anticoagulant is preferred.

CEA is a surgical procedure for the treatment of symptomatic carotid artery disease. Symptomatic patients included those with TIAs, transient monocular blindness, or nondisabling strokes. A meta-analysis by Rothwell et al. of three major randomized controlled trials (the European Carotid Surgery Trial [ECST], the North American Symptomatic Carotid Endarterectomy Trial [NASCET], and the Veterans Affairs Cooperative Study Program [VACS]) showed reduced death or recurrent CVA in patients who underwent CAE for symptomatic carotid stenosis >70% and <99% (Rothwell et al. 2003). These findings have been reproduced in other studies and CEA is a class I recommendation within six months of a TIA or non-disabling CVA for carotid stenosis >70% by angiography (Kernan et al. 2014). This recommendation is based on the assumption that the perioperative risk of CVA and mortality is <6%.

The role of CEA is less clear with symptomatic stenoses in the 50–69% range. Among 858 symptomatic NASCET patients with a stenosis of 50–69%, the 5-year rate of any ipsilateral stroke was 15.7% in patients treated surgically compared with 22.2% in those treated medically ($P = 0.045$). According to the 2014 guidelines, "For patients with recent TIA or ischemic stroke and ipsilateral moderate (50%–69%) carotid stenosis as documented by catheter-based imaging or noninvasive imaging with corroboration (e.g., magnetic resonance angiogram or computed tomography angiogram), CEA is recommended depending on patient-specific factors, such as age, sex, and comorbidities, if the perioperative morbidity and mortality risk is estimated to be <6%" (Kernan et al. 2014).

Carotid artery stenting (CAS) is an endovascular approach to carotid revascularization which holds a similar class I recommendation in the setting of symptomatic carotid stenosis. Patient-specific comorbid conditions and anatomy should be used to help guide which method of revascularization is preferred. In addition, it is a class 3 recommendation to revascularize carotid stenosis <50% or totally occluded carotid arteries. The benefit of revascularization by either modality in asymptomatic carotid stenosis is less clear and currently revascularization in this setting is a 2a recommendation for stenosis >70% (Brott et al. 2011).

Patients Without Atrial Fibrillation or Severe Extracranial or Intracranial Atherosclerosis

The Platelet-Oriented Inhibition in New TIA and Minor Ischemic Stroke (POINT) trial investigated antiplatelet regimens for the prevention of recurrent stroke in patients after TIA or minor stroke (Johnston et al., n.d.). The POINT trial excluded patients with a cardiac source of symptoms such as atrial fibrillation (generally treated with anticoagulation), those with severe extracranial carotid disease (generally treated with CAE or CAS), and those with severe intracranial atherosclerosis (generally treated with dual antiplatelet therapy for three months or longer). Patients were randomly assigned to receive either aspirin (at a dose of 50–325 mg daily) alone or the same dose of aspirin plus clopidogrel (at a dose of 75 mg daily, after a 600-mg loading dose), and treatment was continued for 90 days. The primary outcome was subsequent ischemic stroke, myocardial infarction, or death from ischemic vascular causes.

There were two interesting findings. One, while here was a lower rate of subsequent ischemic events with clopidogrel plus aspirin than with aspirin alone, this was balanced by a higher rate of serious bleeding with the combination. These results are consistent with other trials of combined aspirin plus clopidogrel for stroke prevention after TIA, in which bleeding complications offset lower rates of ischemic events. Second is that most of the benefit regarding stroke prevention occurred in the first week of treatment with the combination, whereas most of the bleeding occurred later. In a secondary analysis, the benefit of aspirin plus clopidogrel in preventing ischemic outcomes was significant during the first 7–30 days of treatment, whereas the risk of major hemorrhage became greater only during the period from 8 to 90 days.

Silent Cerebrovascular Disease

Silent cerebrovascular disease is defined as asymptomatic findings of subcortical cavities or cortical areas of atrophy and gliosis that are presumed to be caused by previous infarction or white matter lesions of presumed vascular origin represent areas of demyelination, gliosis, arteriosclerosis, and microinfarction presumed to be caused by ischemia on brain MRI and CT scans. For patients with silent cerebrovascular disease, the AHA/ASA Scientific Statement suggests "that it may be reasonable to follow AHA/ASA guidelines for primary stroke prevention" (Smith et al. 2017).

References

Barnett, H.J., Taylor, D.W., Eliasziw, M. et al. (1998). Benefit of carotid endarterectomy in patients with symptomatic moderate or severe stenosis. North American Symptomatic Carotid Endarterectomy Trial Collaborators. *The New England Journal of Medicine* 339 (20): 1415–1425. [PubMed: 9811916].

Benjamin, E.J., Virani, S.S., Callaway, C.W. et al. (2010). Heart disease and stroke statistics-2010 update: a report from the American Heart Association. *Circulation* 12 (1): e46–e215.

Brott, T.G., Halperin, J.L., Abbara, S. et al. (2011). 2011 ASA/ACCF/AHA/AANN/AANS/ACR/ASNR/CNS/ SAIP/SCAI/SIR/

SNIS/SVM/SVS guideline on the management of patients with extracranial carotid and vertebral artery disease. A report of the American College of Cardiology Foundation/American Heart Association Task F. *Circulation* 124 (4): e54–e130. [PubMed: 21282504].

CAPRIE Steering Committee (1996). A randomised, blinded, trial of clopidogrel versus aspirin in patients at risk of ischaemic events (CAPRIE). *Lancet* 348: 1329–1339.

Johnston, S.C., Easton, J.D., Farrant, M. et al. Clopidogrel and aspirin in acute ischemic stroke and high-risk TIA. *The New England Journal of Medicine* https://doi.org/10.1056/NEJMoa1800410.

Kernan, W.N., Ovbiagele, B., Black, H.R. et al. (2014). Guidelines for the prevention of stroke in patients with stroke and transient ischemic attack: a guideline for healthcare professionals from the American Heart Association/American Stroke Association. *Stroke* 45 (7): 2160–2236.

Rothwell, P.M., Eliasziw, M., Gutnikov, S.A. et al. (2003). Analysis of pooled data from the randomised controlled trials of endarterectomy for symptomatic carotid stenosis. *Lancet* 361 (9352): 107–116.

Smith, E.E., Saposnik, G., Biessels, G.J. et al. (2017). Prevention of stroke in patients with silent cerebrovascular disease: a scientific statement for healthcare professionals from the American Heart Association/American Stroke Association. *Stroke* 48 (2): e44–e71.

U.S. Preventive Services Task Force. Final Recommendation Statement: Carotid Artery Stenosis: Screening. December 2016. https://www.uspreventiveservicestaskforce.org/Page/Document/Recommendation StatementFinal/carotid-artery-stenosis-screening.

Wityk, R.J., Lehman, D., Klag, M. et al. (1996). Race and sex differences in the distribution of cerebral atherosclerosis. *Stroke* 27 (11): 1974–1980. [PubMed: 8898801].

Case 5: A 54-Year-Old Woman with Exertional Angina But No Atherosclerotic Coronary Artery Disease

A 54-year-old female was referred for cardiology evaluation after reporting a three-hour episode of pressure-like chest pain with radiation to her back that occurred at rest. Past medical history was significant for end-stage renal disease (with a history of a failed kidney transplant) currently treated with hemodialysis, ulcerative colitis status post ileostomy, and prior venous thromboembolic disease. Vital signs showed a heart rate of 95 bpm and blood pressure of 92/55 mmHg. Cardiac and pulmonary examinations were normal.

You order a transthoracic echocardiogram and a stress test. The echocardiogram demonstrated mild left ventricular hypertrophy with hyperdynamic contraction and no focal wall motion abnormalities. The end-systolic volume was small with an estimated left ventricular ejection fraction of greater than 70%.

A dynamic mid-ventricular pressure gradient was observed with a peak outflow velocity in excess of 3.0 m/s. An adenosine technetium-99 m (^{99m}Tc) tetrofosmin myocardial perfusion study revealed a severe, large, dense defect in the mid to distal anterior wall that was predominantly fixed with partial reversibility. Global left ventricular systolic function was normal with ejection fraction of greater than 75% at both rest and stress. Adenosine ^{99m}Tc-tetrofosmin myocardial perfusion imaging performed nearly one year prior, as part of an evaluation for possible repeat renal transplant, had revealed homogenous radioisotrope tracer uptake with no stress-induced perfusion abnormalities.

Angiography of the left coronary artery in an AP cranial projection is shown below (Figure 5.1). What is the diagnosis?

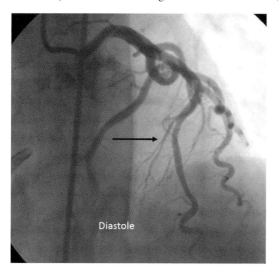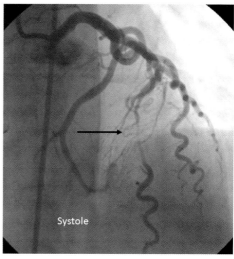

Figure 5.1 Angiography of the left coronary artery in an AP cranial projection.

Cardiology Board Review: ECG, Hemodynamic and Angiographic Unknowns, First Edition. Edited by George A. Stouffer.
© 2019 John Wiley & Sons Ltd. Published 2019 by John Wiley & Sons Ltd.

Myocardial Bridging

Angiography was notable for a large segment of myocardial bridging in the mid-left anterior descending (LAD) coronary artery extending approximately 29 mm with nearly complete lumen obliteration during systole. There was no angiographically significant atherosclerotic coronary artery disease. At the time of the coronary angiography, systemic blood pressure was 80/51 mmHg (mean arterial pressure of 62 mmHg) and the left ventricular end-diastolic pressure (LVEDP) was 1 mmHg.

The patient was encouraged to remain hydrated and started on beta blocker therapy. She had no recurrence of chest pain and a repeat stress test one month later showed normal myocardial perfusion.

Myocardial bridging is an inborn coronary abnormality and is defined as a segment of a major epicardial coronary artery that is located intramurally in the myocardium (Alegria et al. 2005; Angelini et al. 1983; Tarantini et al. 2016). In clinical practice, this term is used to describe an angiographic entity for which the coronary artery narrows during systole (Angelini et al. 1983). While myocardial bridging can occur in any artery, >95% of patients will have involvement of the LAD (Geiringer 1951).

The estimated prevalence of myocardial bridging is 1.5–16% when assessed by coronary angiography, though on autopsy intramyocardial sections of one or more coronary arteries has been found in as many as 80% of people in some studies (Alegria et al. 2005; Geiringer 1951; Tarantini et al. 2016). The existence of many superficial intramuscular segments that are not compressed during systole and thus not visible on angiography. Additionally, myocardial bridging is a dynamic process. Factors influencing the degree of myocardial bridging and thus identification at the time of angiogram include the contractile state of the myocardium, length and thickness of the myocardial bridge, heart rate, blood pressure, and left ventricular preload.

Hemodynamic effects associated with myocardial bridging include (i) increased diastolic velocities; (ii) intracoronary systolic pressure overshooting within the bridge segment; and (iii) reduced coronary flow reserve (CFR). Intracoronary flow within intramyocardial coronary segments typically shows acceleration in early diastole followed by marked deceleration to a plateau in velocity in mid to late diastole in nearly 90% of patients. While the most prominent feature on angiography is systolic compression of the artery, delayed diastolic relaxation and abnormal diastolic flow are also important effects of significant myocardial bridging. Diastolic abnormalities, rather than systolic compression, are important in the development of myocardial ischemia as approximately 85% of coronary blood flow within the LAD occurs within diastole.

The presence of tachycardia may make a myocardial bridge significant by shortening the diastolic period and increasing the importance of systolic blood flow (Schwarz et al. 1996). Schwarz et al. investigated this theory by utilizing atrial pacing to induce tachycardia in patients with an angiographically proven myocardial bridge of the LAD. They discovered that there was luminal narrowing of 84% during systole with persistent decrease in arterial diameter during diastole. This effect in both systole and diastole was mitigated substantially by administration of intravenous beta blockade, which was also associated with a decrease in anginal symptoms (Schwarz et al. 1996). Alternatively, myocardial bridging has been thought to cause acute coronary syndromes (ACS) by systolic kinking of blood vessels, especially at high heart rates, thus causing damaged endothelium which leads to ACS (Ciampricotti and el Gamal 1988; Gertz et al. 1981). Another potential mechanism of myocardial ischemia at the site of a myocardial bridge is the development of concurrent atherosclerosis which usually occurs at the beginning or end of the bridging segment due to turbulent flow.

Myocardial bridging is particularly common in patients with hypertrophic cardiomyopathy, and has an estimated prevalence of 30% in this population (Kitazume et al. 1983). Compared to patients with hypertrophic cardiomyopathy without bridging, those with bridging had higher frequency of chest pain, cardiac arrest, ventricular tachycardia, reduction in systolic blood pressure during exercise, more ST-segment depression with exercise, and a greater degree of dispersion of the corrected QT interval (Alegria et al. 2005). Interestingly, it is not clear that survival is affected by the presence of myocardial bridging, and various studies have had conflicting findings (Alegria et al. 2005; Sorajja et al. 2003).

Optimal treatment of myocardial bridging has yet to be determined by randomized controlled trials (Tarantini et al. 2016). As discussed above, beta blockers decrease tachycardia and increase diastolic filling time of the coronary arteries, and therefore these agents are thought to be beneficial (Schwarz et al. 1996). The utilization of bare metal stents has been associated with high rates of restenosis. Haager et al. found that at seven weeks approximately 50% of patients had at least mild to moderate in-stent stenosis, with a large portion of these patients needing repeat revascularization (Haager et al. 2000). Clinical outcomes with drug eluting stents are better but there is not sufficient data to make compelling recommendations. While one study has shown that stenting can decrease hemodynamic abnormalities and improve symptoms (Klues et al. 1997), no study has consistently shown normalization of perfusion defects that were present before stent implantation. Patients can be treated with myotomy but surgical treatment should be limited to patients with symptoms that persist despite appropriate medical therapy. Outcomes are good when the procedure is performed by an experienced surgeon (Katznelson et al. 1996).

References

Alegria, J.R., Herrmann, J., Holmes, D.R. Jr. et al. (2005). Myocardial bridging. *European Heart Journal* 26 (12): 1159–1168.

Angelini, P., Trivellato, M., Donis, J. et al. (1983). Myocardial bridges: a review. *Progress in Cardiovascular Diseases* 26 (1): 75–88.

Ciampricotti, R. and el Gamal, M. (1988). Vasospastic coronary occlusion associated with a myocardial bridge. *Catheterization and Cardiovascular Diagnosis* 14 (2): 118–120.

Geiringer, E. (1951). The mural coronary. *American Heart Journal* 41 (3): 359–368.

Gertz, S.D., Uretsky, G., Wajnberg, R.S. et al. (1981). Endothelial cell damage and thrombus formation after partial arterial constriction: relevance to the role of coronary artery spasm in the pathogenesis of myocardial infarction. *Circulation* 63 (3): 476–486.

Haager, P.K., Schwarz, E.R., vom Dahl, J. et al. (2000). Long term angiographic and clinical follow up in patients with stent implantation for symptomatic myocardial bridging. *Heart* 84 (4): 403–408.

Katznelson, Y., Petchenko, P., Knobel, B. et al. (1996). Myocardial bridging: surgical technique and operative results. *Military Medicine* 161 (4): 248–250.

Kitazume, H., Kramer, J.R., Krauthamer, D. et al. (1983). Myocardial bridges in obstructive hypertrophic cardiomyopathy. *American Heart Journal* 106 (1 Pt 1): 131–135.

Klues, H.G., Schwarz, E.R., vom Dahl, J. et al. (1997). Disturbed intracoronary hemodynamics in myocardial bridging: early normalization by intracoronary stent placement. *Circulation* 96 (9): 2905–2913.

Schwarz, E.R., Klues, H.G., vom Dahl, J. et al. (1996). Functional, angiographic and intracoronary Doppler flow characteristics in symptomatic patients with myocardial bridging: effect of short-term intravenous beta-blocker medication. *Journal of the American College of Cardiology* 27 (7): 1637–1645.

Sorajja, P., Ommen, S.R., Nishimura, R.A. et al. (2003). Myocardial bridging in adult patients with hypertrophic cardiomyopathy. *Journal of the American College of Cardiology* 42 (5): 889–894.

Tarantini, G., Migliore, F., Cademartiri, F. et al. (2016). Left anterior descending artery myocardial bridging: A Clinical Approach. *Journal of the American College of Cardiology* 68 (25): 2887–2899. https://doi.org/10.1016/j. jacc.2016.09.973.

Case 6: A 34-Year-Old Woman with Fatigue

A 34-year-old female with systemic lupus erythematosus (SLE), hypertension, and hypothyroidism is referred to you for evaluation of fatigue. She was diagnosed with SLE five years ago and has been doing well on hydroxychloroquine. Her only other medications are lisinopril and levothyroxine. Her primary complaint is generalized fatigue, such that she is not able to complete her typical daily activities around home without rest. This has progressed over the past year. She does feel shortness of breath if she overexerts herself, but admits she is not particularly active due to fatigue.

On review of systems, she notes unintentional weight loss of 10 pounds over the past year. She feels dizzy if she overexerts herself and has a dry cough particularly in the mornings. She has noted swelling in her feet and legs, to the point where it is difficult to wear her normal shoe size. She has had no chest pain or palpitations.

Physical exam is notable for a heart rate of 90 bpm, blood pressure 149/70 mmHg, and oxygen saturation of 94%. Jugular veins are distended, and jugular venous pressure is estimated at 10 cm H_2O. Cardiac exam shows regular rate and rhythm, prominent S2, and no murmurs. Peripheral pulses are equal and symmetric. She has 2+ pitting edema to mid-shin bilaterally. Lungs are clear.

Laboratory evaluation shows stable low-normal hemoglobin and normal TSH. Renal function is normal.

The ECG is shown in Figure 6.1 and suggests right atrial (RA) enlargement and right

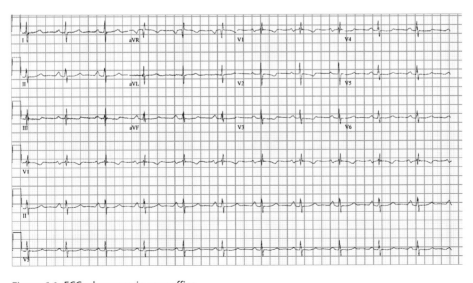

Figure 6.1 ECG when seen in your office.

Cardiology Board Review: ECG, Hemodynamic and Angiographic Unknowns, First Edition. Edited by George A. Stouffer.
© 2019 John Wiley & Sons Ltd. Published 2019 by John Wiley & Sons Ltd.

Table 6.1 Hemodynamic measurements.

Mean right atrial (RA) pressure	12 mmHg
Right ventricular (RV) pressure (systolic/end diastolic)	71/10 mmHg
Pulmonary capillary wedge pressure (PCWP)	10 mmHg
Pulmonary artery (PA) pressure	80/42 mmHg
Mean PA pressure	56 mmHg
Pulmonary vascular resistance (PVR)	13.1
Oxygen saturation in the PA	67%
Cardiac output (CO) by assumed Fick method	3.55 L/min

ventricular hypertrophy (RVH) and has a rightward axis.

An echocardiogram showed normal left ventricular function, an enlarged right ventricle, and RA dilation. Pulmonary artery (PA) pressure could not be accurately estimated due to poor echo windows. No significant valve abnormalities were visualized.

Right heart catheterization (RHC) was performed with hemodynamic measurements as shown in Table 6.1.

What type of pulmonary hypertension does she have according to World Health Organization (WHO) classification? What is the most likely cause of her pulmonary hypertension?

Pulmonary Hypertension

The case describes a 34-year-old woman with SLE who presents for evaluation of fatigue. Physical examination, ECG, and echocardiography are suggestive of right heart failure and right heart catheterization shows severe pulmonary hypertension (PH) (mean PA pressure of 56 mmHg), normal PCWP (pulmonary capillary wedge pressure), and markedly elevated PVR (pulmonary vascular resistance). These findings are diagnostic of PH that is not due to elevated left-heart pressures. As discussed below, the

classification of PH requires evaluation of possible underlying etiologies. The patient could have group 1, 3, 4, or 5 PH and further testing is needed.

Definition of PH and Pathophysiology

The normal pulmonary circulation is a low-resistance vascular bed with the ability to maintain stable perfusion pressures under physiological increases in blood flow due to increased cardiac output (CO). For example, during exercise, recruitment and distension of pulmonary capillaries accommodate increases in CO and prevents significant elevations of right ventricular (RV) afterload and energy consumption. Normal mean pulmonary artery pressure (MPAP) is less than 20 mmHg, varies little with age, and is independent of sex and ethnicity. Chronically increased MPAP is referred to as PH and is defined by a MPAP of 25 mmHg or greater as measured by right heart catheterization.

There are multiple causes of PH, each with their own unique pathological mechanisms. Regardless of the etiology, the effects of elevated PA pressure on the RV are similar (Vonk Noordegraaf et al. 2017). The RV is a high-volume, low-pressure pump and is able to accommodate changes in blood volume better than significant changes in pressure. The RV initially responds to elevated PA pressure by increasing contractility and subsequently by developing hypertrophy. If PA pressure continues to rise above the ability of the RV to increase contractility, the RV begins to dilate in response to increased preload, and heart rate increases. RV dilation initially allows the RV to expand without affecting left ventricle (LV) function. However, as PH progresses, the dilation of the RV produces septal bowing which impedes LV filling. Additionally, oxygen demand by the RV increases as a result of increased contractility, geometric remodeling, and increased heart rate. At the end-stage of PH, inefficient interventricular interaction and increased metabolic demand ultimately lead to both RV and LV failure.

Classification of PH

PH is not a single disease but instead reflects a large number of clinical entities which each have their own unique pathophysiology and natural history. The WHO classification system organizes PH into five categories based on underlying mechanisms (Table 6.2) (Simonneau et al. 2013).

Table 6.2 WHO Classification of PH.

Group 1. Pulmonary arterial hypertension (PAH)
Idiopathic PAH
Heritable PAH
Drug and toxin-induced
Associated with connective tissue diseases, HIV, congenital heart disease, portal hypertension, Schistosomiasis
Pulmonary veno-occlusive disease

Group 2. PH caused by left-sided heart disease
Heart failure with reduced ejection fraction (HFrEF)
Heart failure with preserved ejection fraction (HFpEF)
Valvular disease
Congenital/acquired left-sided inflow/outflow tract obstruction

Group 3. PH caused by lung diseases and/or hypoxia
Chronic obstructive pulmonary disease
Interstitial lung disease
Sleep-related disordered breathing
Alveolar hypoventilation disorders
Chronic high-altitude exposure

Group 4. Chronic thromboembolic pulmonary hypertension (CTEPH)

Group 5. PH with unclear and/or multifactorial mechanisms
Hematologic disorders: chronic hemolytic anemia, myeloproliferative disorders
Systemic disorders: sarcoidosis, pulmonary Langerhans cell histiocytosis, vasculitis
Metabolic disorders: thyroid disease, glycogen storage disease, Gaucher disease
Chronic kidney disease

PH = pulmonary hypertension.
Source: Table is modified from Simonneau et al. (2013).

Group 1 encompasses idiopathic, heritable, and acquired etiologies in which the primary source of pathology is medial hyperplasia in the distal pulmonary arteries. A rare cause of Group 1 PH is pulmonary veno-occlusive disease due to obliteration of the small pulmonary venules, as well as distal arterial hypertrophy and fibrosis (Montani et al. 2016). PH associated with connective tissue disorders, most commonly scleroderma, is included in Group 1. Additionally, congenital heart disease resulting in systemic to pulmonary shunting of blood and subsequent PH (typified by Eisenmenger's syndrome) is included in Group 1.

Group 2 includes PH due to elevated left-sided filling pressures. Increased left-sided filling pressures, as reflected by elevated PCWP or LV end-diastolic pressure (LVEDP), result in passive backward transmission of pressure through the pulmonary veins and subsequently the capillary bed. Pathologically, this results in thickened pulmonary veins, dilated capillaries, and interstitial edema. Unlike Group 1 PH, the distal pulmonary arteries of patients with Group 2 PH often do not have medial hypertrophy or intimal fibrosis. Therefore, PVR and the transpulmonary gradient (TPG) are both typically normal; elevated levels would indicate PH that is "out of proportion" to that expected from elevated left-atrial pressure alone. This may reflect a reactive vasoconstriction of the distal pulmonary arterioles due to prolonged or more severe left-sided heart disease.

Group 3 includes PH caused by chronic respiratory disease and chronic hypoxia. The pulmonary arterioles are unique in that they vasoconstrict due to hypoxia. This is an important mechanism which allows for the careful balance of perfusion and ventilation in the case of localized alveolar hypoxia (Aaronson et al. 2006). However, in response to sustained hypoxia, this regulatory mechanism becomes detrimental and results in pathological arterial remodeling. Furthermore, diseases which affect the lung interstitium result in chronic inflammation and loss of pulmonary capillaries, further exacerbating the pathological remodeling due to hypoxia. Long-term oxygen therapy and smoking cessation are important components of therapy and may result in stabilization or even attenuation of PH in some patients.

Group 4 is chronic thromboembolic pulmonary hypertension (CTEPH) and is defined as PH occurring coincident with a segmental perfusion defect on lung imaging, despite three months of effective anticoagulation, and in the absence of elevated left-heart filling pressures. CTEPH occurs as a result of venous pulmonary thromboembolism and inadequate resolution of clot formation (Simonneau et al. 2017). Why this occurs in some people with pulmonary embolism and not others is unclear. CTEPH is potentially treatable with surgery (pulmonary thromboendarterectomy) or percutaneous treatments although outcomes vary widely depending on center experience.

Group 5 includes etiologies with either multifactorial or unclear mechanisms. For example, sickle cell disease and subsequent hemolytic anemia can lead to PH via high-output heart failure, recurrent microthrombosis, and hypoxia. Sarcoidosis may result in PH via multiple mechanisms due to the tendency of granulomatous infiltration to affect the pulmonary vasculature, lung parenchyma, and the myocardium. Other rare causes of PH are also shown in Table 6.2.

Clinical Evaluation

The most common presenting symptoms of PH include exertional dyspnea, reduced exercise tolerance, and fatigue. Additional symptoms include chest pain, syncope with exertion, and lower extremity edema owing to RV failure in more advanced disease. On physical exam, patients commonly have elevated jugular venous pressure with prominent A waves due to the contraction of the right atrium against a non-compliant, hypertrophied RV. Contraction of the hypertrophied RV may be palpated as a parasternal

heave. Auscultation often reveals a prominent pulmonary component of S2 due to the increased force of pulmonic valve closure in the presence of elevated PA pressure. In more advanced PH, murmurs associated with tricuspid and pulmonary valve insufficiency (Graham Steele murmur – an early diastolic decrescendo murmur) may be heard. Tricuspid insufficiency results in a holosystolic murmur that increases with inspiration and is best heard at the left lower sternal border. Pulmonary valve regurgitation results in an early diastolic decrescendo murmur at the left upper sternal border.

ECG findings consistent with PH are nonspecific but are consistent with the pathophysiology and include right axis deviation, RA enlargement, and RV hypertrophy with strain. Common arrhythmias include sinus tachycardia, focal or multifocal atrial tachycardia, and atrial flutter.

The evaluation of a patient with symptoms suggestive of PH begins with echocardiography with Doppler which allows non-invasive estimation of PA pressure and assessment of right heart remodeling and function (Rudski et al. 2010). Furthermore, echocardiography allows evaluation of contributing factors for PH development and for processes with similar clinical presentations including cardiomyopathies, valvular disease, pericardial effusions, and intracardiac shunt. Assuming that no gradient exists across the RV outflow tract due to congenital disease or pulmonary valve stenosis, RV systolic pressure (RVSP) is approximately equal to systolic PA pressure (SPAP). RVSP can be estimated using the modified Bernoulli equation: $RVSP = 4v^2 + RA$ pressure, where "v" is peak tricuspid regurgitation (TR) jet velocity and RA pressure is estimated from the echocardiographic assessment of the IVC. It is important to note that the echocardiographic estimate of SPAP should be interpreted in the context of an individual patient's clinical presentation, past medical history, and other echocardiography findings which together allow an assessment of the probability of PH (Galie et al. 2016). It is generally accepted that estimated SPAP

>40 mmHg in the absence of left-sided heart disease or lung disease warrants confirmation of PH by RHC and evaluation for causes of Group 1 PH.

RHC is necessary to confirm the diagnosis of PH, defined as a MPAP >25 mmHg, and evaluate the contribution of left-sided heart disease to elevated PA pressure, by measurement of PCWP. PCWP is used as a surrogate for left atrial pressure, with values <15 mmHg indicating normal left-heart filling pressure. Direct measurement of pressures with left heart catheterization with or without coronary angiography may be pursued in some cases depending on clinical history. Suspicion for ischemic heart disease, echocardiography consistent with cardiomyopathy or structural disease, or technically difficult PCWP measurements all warrant further testing.

CO, TPG, and PVR are important calculated parameters helpful in the evaluation of PH. CO can be calculated from PA and venous oxygen saturation using the Fick method or by thermodilution. TPG = MPAP – PCWP and is normally <12 mmHg. PVR = TPG/CO and is normally <3 Wood units (or < 240 dynes-sec/cm^{-5}). Determination of the primary etiology for PH is critical to guide therapy, as those with Group 1 PH benefit from pulmonary vasodilators whereas those with other forms of PH may have no benefit or even be harmed by these therapies. As shown in Table 6.3, the diagnosis of Group 1 PH requires a PCWP <15 mmHg with elevated TPG and PVR. Elevated TPG and PVR in the setting of PCWP ≥15 mmHg may be due to pulmonary arterial and capillary vasoconstriction and remodeling in response to longstanding or severe elevations in left heart pressures (Rosenkranz et al. 2016).

RHC is not only critical for diagnosis of PH but is also useful to guide management decisions and for prognostication, particularly in patients with Group 1 PH (Barst et al. 2009; Galie et al. 2016). For example, a patient with severely elevated PA pressure, evidence of RV failure with high RA pressures, and low CO may need aggressive treatment with multiple agents whereas a more conservative approach may be taken in a patient with modest PA pressure elevation without evidence of RV failure. Measurement of RA pressure and PCWP allows for quantitative assessment of volume status and is helpful in guiding diuresis. Vasodilator testing during RHC when there is evidence of Group 1 PH should be performed to guide therapy. A robust response to vasodilator is defined by a decrease in mean PA pressure > 10 mmHg and indicates a high probability of successful treatment with vasodilator therapy beginning with calcium channel blockers. Vasodilators used in the catheterization lab include intravenous calcium channel blockers, adenosine, epoprostenal, or inhaled nitric oxide. Volume loading may also be used in the catheterization lab to distinguish Group 1 PH vs Group 2 PH due to heart failure with preserved ejection fraction (HFpEF). In patients where HFpEF is suspected, but without elevated PWCP, a small volume load may unmask elevated filling pressures.

Table 6.3 Distinguishing Group 1 (PAH) and Group 2 (HF) by hemodynamic parameters.

	Normal	Group 1 (PAH)	Group 2 (HF)	PH "out of proportion" to HF alone
PA mean (mmHg)	<25	≥25	Normal or ≥25	≥25
PCWP (mmHg)	≤12	≤15	>15	>15
TPG (mmHg)	≤12	>12	Normal	>12
PVR (Wood units)	≤3	>3	Normal	>3

PA = pulmonary artery; PCWP = pulmonary capillary wedge pressure; TPG = transpulmonary gradient (mean PA – mean PCWP); PVR = pulmonary vascular resistance.

Treatment

Treatment of PH is highly dependent on the etiology as defined by the WHO Group (Galie et al. 2016; McLaughlin et al. 2009). Patients with group 2–5 PH should have aggressive treatment of the underlying condition. The use of diuretics is a common link between all forms of PH, although diuretics should be used cautiously to avoid excessive reduction of RV preload. Calcium channel blockers are useful in Group 1 PH with reversibility on vasodilator testing. Patients with Group 1 PH may also benefit from phosphodiesterase type V inhibitors, endothelin receptor antagonists, and prostacyclin analogues (Maron and Galie 2016).

References

Aaronson, P.I., Robertson, T.P., Knock, G.A. et al. (2006). Hypoxic pulmonary vasoconstriction: mechanisms and controversies. *The Journal of Physiology* 570 (Pt 1): 53–58. https://doi.org/10.1113/jphysiol.2005.098855. Epub 2005 Oct 27.

Barst, R.J., Gibbs, J.S., Ghofrani, H.A. et al. (2009). Updated evidence-based treatment algorithm in pulmonary arterial hypertension. *Journal of the American College of Cardiology* 54 (1 Suppl): S78–S84. https://doi.org/10.1016/j.jacc.2009.04.017.

Galie, N., Humbert, M., Vachiery, J.L. et al. (2016). 2015 ESC/ERS Guidelines for the diagnosis and treatment of pulmonary hypertension: The joint task force for the diagnosis and treatment of pulmonary hypertension of the European Society of Cardiology (ESC) and the European Respiratory Society (ERS): Endorsed by: Association for European Paediatric and Congenital Cardiology (AEPC), International Society for Heart and Lung Transplantation (ISHLT). *European Heart Journal* 37 (1): 67–119. https://doi.org/10.1093/eurheartj/ehv317. Epub 2015 Aug 29.

Maron, B.A. and Galie, N. (2016). Diagnosis, treatment, and clinical management of pulmonary arterial hypertension in the contemporary era: a review. *JAMA Cardiology* 1 (9): 1056–1065. https://doi.org/10.1001/jamacardio.2016.4471.

McLaughlin, V.V., Badesch, D.B., Delcroix, M. et al. (2009). End points and clinical trial design in pulmonary arterial hypertension. *Journal of the American College of Cardiology* 54 (1 Suppl): S97–S107. https://doi.org/10.1016/j.jacc.2009.04.007.

Montani, D., Lau, E.M., Dorfmuller, P. et al. (2016). Pulmonary veno-occlusive disease. *The European Respiratory Journal* 47 (5): 1518–1534. https://doi.org/10.1183/13993003.00026-2016. Epub 2016 Mar 23.

Rosenkranz, S., Gibbs, J.S., Wachter, R. et al. (2016). Left ventricular heart failure and pulmonary hypertension. *European Heart Journal* 37 (12): 942–954. https://doi.org/10.1093/eurheartj/ehv512. Epub 2015 Oct 27.

Rudski, L.G., Lai, W.W., Afilalo, J. et al. (2010). Guidelines for the echocardiographic assessment of the right heart in adults: a report from the American Society of Echocardiography endorsed by the European Association of Echocardiography, a registered branch of the European Society of Cardiology, and the Canadian Society of Echocardiography. *Journal of the American Society of Echocardiography* 23 (7): 685–713; quiz 786–788. https://doi: org/10.1016/j.echo.2010.05.010.

Simonneau, G., Gatzoulis, M.A., Adatia, I. et al. (2013). Updated clinical classification of pulmonary hypertension. *Journal of the American College of Cardiology* 62 (25

Suppl): D34–D41. https://doi.org/10.1016/j. jacc.2013.10.029.

Simonneau, G., Torbicki, A., Dorfmuller, P. et al. (2017). The pathophysiology of chronic thromboembolic pulmonary hypertension. *European Respiratory Review* 26 (143): pii: p. 26/143/160112. https://doi.org/10.1183/16000617.0112-2016. Print 2017 Mar 31.

Vonk Noordegraaf, A., Westerhof, B.E., and Westerhof, N. (2017). The relationship between the right ventricle and its load in pulmonary hypertension. *Journal of the American College of Cardiology* 69 (2): 236–243. https://doi.org/10.1016/j. jacc.2016.10.047.

Case 7: An Elderly Woman with a Loud Murmur

You are referred a 76-year-old female because her primary care provider heard a loud murmur. She has a past medical history of pulmonary stenosis treated with surgical pulmonary valvotomy as a child, coronary artery disease, chronic atrial fibrillation, chronic obstructive lung disease, hypertension, type 2 diabetes mellitus, renal artery stenosis, and stage 3 chronic kidney disease. Her major complaints are dyspnea on exertion and lower extremity edema. She denied any chest pain. On cardiac auscultation, she was noted to have an irregularly irregular rhythm w/regular rate, a IV/VI systolic murmur heard best at the left sternal border, and a III/VI diastolic murmur heard best at the left lower sternal border. Her examination was also notable for a right ventricular (RV) heave, jugular venous distention, coarse breath sounds on lung examination, and 1+ lower extremity edema bilaterally.

Transthoracic echocardiography (TTE) showed a normal left ventricular ejection fraction (65–70%), moderate pulmonary regurgitation, RV hypertrophy, moderate tricuspid regurgitation (TR), dilated right ventricle, and dilated right atrium.

A right heart catheterization was performed and the following pulmonary artery (PA) pressure tracing obtained (Figure 7.1).

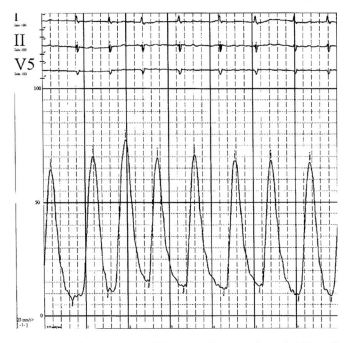

Figure 7.1 Pulmonary artery (PA) pressure (measured on a 0–100 mmHg scale).

Cardiology Board Review: ECG, Hemodynamic and Angiographic Unknowns, First Edition. Edited by George A. Stouffer.
© 2019 John Wiley & Sons Ltd. Published 2019 by John Wiley & Sons Ltd.

What is the most likely cause of her dyspnea and lower extremity edema?

Pulmonic Regurgitation

Note that the PA diastolic pressure is very low (~10 mmHg) and PA systolic pressure is elevated (consistent with increased flow across the pulmonic valve). This is consistent with severe pulmonic regurgitation (PR). This is confirmed by simultaneous measurement of PA and RV waveforms which demonstrates that they are similar in configuration (Figure 7.2).

Background

Mild PR is a common occurrence in many healthy individuals. However, more severe cases of PR may result from various disor-

ders. These cases can lead to RV volume overload and right-sided heart failure.

Etiology and Pathogenesis

The etiologies of PR can be classified into physiologic, primary, and secondary causes. Physiologic trivial or mild PR is a common finding on Doppler echocardiography in many healthy individuals (Yoshida et al. 1988). Primary valvular causes of significant PR include iatrogenic, infectious, immune-mediated, systemic, and congenital conditions. This category includes diseases such as endocarditis, rheumatic heart disease, carcinoid syndrome, and Marfan's syndrome. Secondary PR occurs in patients with morphologically normal pulmonic valves who have severe pulmonary hypertension (either primary or secondary), PA dilation, or both (Goins et al. 2018).

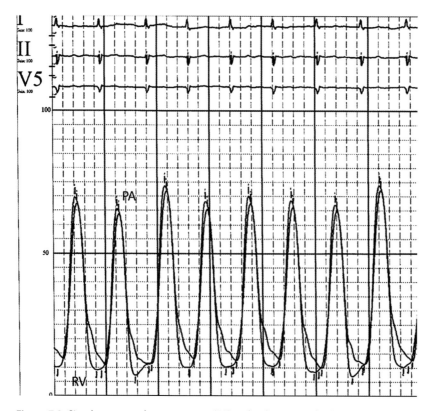

Figure 7.2 Simultaneous pulmonary artery (PA) and right ventricular (RV) pressures in the patient described in the case on a 0 – 100 mmHg scale.

The most common cause of PR is iatrogenic, due to surgical valvotomy or balloon pulmonary valvuloplasty (McCrindle and Kan 1991). These procedures are performed for RV outflow obstruction due to Tetralogy of Fallot or congenital pulmonic valve stenosis. Over time, PR can develop in these patients.

Clinical Presentation

Patients with PR are often asymptomatic prior to the development of RV dysfunction. As the condition progresses, patients with severe PR may eventually present with signs and symptoms of right-sided heart failure. Initial symptoms may include dyspnea and fatigue, and less commonly palpitations, lightheadedness, and syncope. Atrial and ventricular arrhythmias can occur as the condition progresses. Patients with isolated severe PR seldom present with chest pain.

Findings on physical examination vary depending on the severity and cause of the PR. The characteristic physical finding of PR is a decrescendo diastolic murmur, loudest at the left third and fourth intercostal spaces, which increases with inspiration. Typically, S2 will be widely split. The pulmonic component may be accentuated if there is significant pulmonary hypertension. Patients may have a high-pitched and "blowing" diastolic murmur with a prominent P2 in the presence of severe pulmonary hypertension, which is known as the classic Graham Steell murmur. If there is no significant pulmonary hypertension, then the murmur will be low-pitched, which is less commonly found. Occasionally, patients will present with an associated crescendo-decrescendo systolic murmur from increased flow across the pulmonary valve or a holosystolic murmur due to coincident tricuspid regurgitation. Jugular venous distension and other signs of right-sided heart failure may also be noted on physical examination (Goins et al. 2018).

Diagnosis and Management

TTE with Doppler is very important in the diagnosis of patients with pulmonary regurgitation. These patients often also have an electrocardiogram (ECG) and chest x-ray, although these are not required for the diagnosis. The ECG in patients with pulmonary regurgitation may show evidence of right-axis deviation and RV hypertrophy. Chest x-ray may show evidence of RV enlargement and may also show right atrial enlargement if co-existing tricuspid regurgitation is also present.

TTE with Doppler imaging can be used to assess the severity of the PR and assess for associated complications, including RV enlargement, decreased RV function, and TR. Parasternal short and long axis windows are ideal for visualizing the pulmonic valve on echocardiography. The severity of PR is determined by the jet width and jet duration. Mild PR is classified by a thin regurgitant jet, while moderate PR is classified by a wider regurgitant jet that remains <50% of the width of the pulmonic valve annulus. Severe PR is classified by the presence of a regurgitant jet that fills >50% of the width of the pulmonary valve annulus. Typically, the regurgitant jet seen in PR is holosystolic. However, if the PR is severe enough, the PA and RV pressures may equalize during early-to-mid diastole causing termination of the jet (Baumgartner et al. 2010; Goins et al. 2018; Nishimura et al. 2014; Warnes et al. 2008). Distorted leaflets, absent leaflets, and annular dilatation may also be seen on TTE in patients with PR (Nishimura et al. 2014).

Mild to moderate PR found on echocardiography is common and does not require intervention or follow-up if the patient is asymptomatic without RV dysfunction or dilatation. Surgical pulmonary valve replacement is indicated in patients with severe, symptomatic PR (Warnes et al. 2008). Surgical replacement is also indicated if the patient has asymptomatic PR with progressive right heart failure (Baumgartner et al. 2010). The goal of valve replacement is to reduce damage to the right ventricle from volume overload. If the patient has secondary PR, medical therapy should be directed toward treating the underlying cause of the PR, for example pulmonary hypertension (Nishimura et al. 2014; Warnes et al. 2008).

A pulmonic valve can be implanted percutaneously as a nonsurgical treatment for patients with right ventricular outflow tract (RVOT) conduit dysfunction. These valves are intended for use in a failing and dysfunctional (stenotic or regurgitant) right ventricle-to-pulmonary artery conduit (most commonly placed during surgery for Tetralogy of Fallot).

Percutaneous intervention is recommended in symptomatic patients with RV systolic pressure >60 mmHg and/or moderate to severe PR and is suggested in asymptomatic patients with severe RVOT obstruction and/or severe PR with at least one of the following criteria – (a) Decrease in exercise capacity on cardiopulmonary exercise testing; (b) Progressive RV dilation; (c) Progressive RV systolic dysfunction; (d) Progressive TR (at least moderate); (e) RV systolic pressure >80 mmHg (TR velocity > 4.3 m/s); or (f) Sustained atrial/ventricular arrhythmias.

References

Baumgartner, H., Bonhoeffer, P., De Groot, N.M.S. et al. (2010). ESC guidelines for the management of grown-up congenital heart disease (new version 2010) the Task Force on the Management of Grown-up Congenital Heart Disease of the European Society of Cardiology (ESC). *European Heart Journal* 31 (23): 2915–2957.

Goins, A., Tate, D.A., and Stouffer, G.A. (2018). Tricuspid and pulmonic valve disease. In: *Netter Cardiology*, 3e (ed. G. Stouffer, M.S. Runge, C. Patterson and J. Rossi), 336–340. Philadelphia PA. Chapter 48: Elsevier.

McCrindle, B.W. and Kan, J.S. (1991). Long-term results after balloon pulmonary valvuloplasty. *Circulation* 83: 1915.

Nishimura, R.A., Otto, C.M., Bonow, R.O. et al. (2014). 2014 AHA/ACC guideline for the management of patients with valvular heart disease: a report of the American College of Cardiology/American Heart Association Task Force on Practice Guidelines. *Journal of the American College of Cardiology* 63 (22): e57–e185.

Warnes, C.A., Williams, R.G., Bashore, T.M. et al. (2008). ACC/AHA 2008 guidelines for the Management of Adults with congenital heart disease: executive summary: a report of the American College of Cardiology/American Heart Association Task Force on Practice Guidelines (writing committee to develop guidelines for the management of adults with congenital heart disease). *Circulation* 118: 2395–2451.

Yoshida, K., Yoshikawa, J., Shakudo, M. et al. (1988). Color Doppler evaluation of valvular regurgitation in normal subjects. *Circulation* 78: 840.

Case 8: A Middle-Aged Woman Who Passes out While Running after her Grandchildren

You are asked to see a 52-year-old female who reported to her primary care provider that she had "passed out." The syncope occurred while she was running upstairs after a grandchild. She also reports worsening dyspnea on exertion.

On physical examination, her blood pressure is 125/74 mmHg, heart rate is 70 bpm, and oxygen saturation is 98% on room air. Her cardiovascular examination is remarkable for a loud systolic murmur heard best at the left upper sternal border which varies in intensity with respiration. You make a tentative diagnosis of pulmonic valve stenosis which is confirmed on echocardiogram with a peak instantaneous gradient of 40 mmHg and mean gradient of 21 mmHg.

Would this patient meet the guidelines for pulmonary valve intervention?

Pulmonic Stenosis

This patient would meet criteria for pulmonary valvuloplasty according to the 2018 American College of Cardiology/American Heart Association (ACC/AHA) Guideline for the Management of Adults with Congenital Heart Disease. The 2018 ACC/AHA Congenital Heart guidelines define the severity of pulmonic stenosis (PS) based on echo-derived velocity across the valve determined using continuous wave Doppler. Mild, moderate, and severe are defined as peak gradient <36 mmHg, 36–64 mmHg, and >64 mmHg, respectively. Balloon valvuloplasty is a class 1

recommendation for patients with moderate or severe PS who have "otherwise unexplained symptoms of HF, cyanosis from interatrial right-to-left communication, and/or exercise intolerance." Asymptomatic patients with a peak gradient <36 mmHg should have a follow-up physical examination, TTE with Doppler, and ECG every five years and asymptomatic patients with peak gradient 36–64 mmHg should have follow-up every two years (Table 8.1). More severe PS needs more frequent follow-up, preferably with an Adult with Congenital Heart Disease specialist. Surgical therapy is recommended for patients with severe PS who are not good candidates for balloon valvuloplasty, e.g. with a hypoplastic pulmonary annulus, severe pulmonary regurgitation, subvalvular PS, or supravalvular PS. Surgical therapy is preferred for most cases of dysplastic pulmonic valve or if severe tricuspid regurgitation is present in addition to the PS.

Background

Stenosis of the pulmonic valve is a relatively common congenital defect, with an incidence rate of approximately 10% in children with congenital heart disease. It is typically associated with a benign clinical course, and in cases of more severe right ventricular outflow obstruction, excellent treatment options are available. Thus, the condition has a very high rate of survival into adulthood.

Cardiology Board Review: ECG, Hemodynamic and Angiographic Unknowns, First Edition. Edited by George A. Stouffer.
© 2019 John Wiley & Sons Ltd. Published 2019 by John Wiley & Sons Ltd.

Table 8.1 AHA/ACC Congenital Heart Disease Guidelines definition of physiologic class and follow-up for PS.

Physiologic state	Characteristics	Follow-up for PS (months)
A	• NYHA FC I symptoms • No hemodynamic or anatomic sequelae • No arrhythmias • Normal exercise capacity • Normal renal/hepatic/pulmonary function	36–60
B	• NYHA FC II symptoms • Mild hemodynamic sequelae (mild aortic enlargement, mild ventricular enlargement, mild ventricular dysfunction) • Mild valvular disease • Trivial or small shunt (not hemodynamically significant) • Arrhythmia not requiring treatment • Abnormal objective cardiac limitation to exercise	24
C	• NYHA FC III symptoms • Significant (moderate or greater) valvular disease; moderate or greater ventricular dysfunction (systemic, pulmonic, or both) • Moderate aortic enlargement • Venous or arterial stenosis • Mild or moderate hypoxemia/cyanosis • Hemodynamically significant shunt • Arrhythmias controlled with treatment • Pulmonary hypertension (less than severe) • End-organ dysfunction responsive to therapy	6–12
D	• NYHA FC IV symptoms • Severe aortic enlargement • Arrhythmias refractory to treatment • Severe hypoxemia (almost always associated with cyanosis) • Severe pulmonary hypertension • Eisenmenger syndrome • Refractory end-organ dysfunction	3–6

NYHA FC = New York Heart Association functional class.

Etiology and Pathogenesis

PS can occur in the following three locations: subvalvular, valvular, or supravalvular. Subvalvular PS consists of a fibromuscular narrowing that is limited to the right ventricular outflow tract. Supravalvular PS, on the other hand, involves an isolated area or multiple areas of narrowing of the main pulmonary artery or branches. Both the subvalvular and supravalvular forms are usually associated with other congenital heart disease, such as Tetralogy of Fallot and the congenital rubella syndrome.

True valvular PS usually occurs as an isolated condition. It may occur as the sole cardiac abnormality in patients with Noonan's syndrome. PS will present with varying degrees of fibrous thickening and fusion of the commissures. In PS, pulmonary artery dilation may be present due to underlying connective tissue abnormality and/or eccentric flow as a consequence of the stenotic valve. In severe cases, right ventricular hypertrophy may also develop over time. Rarely, PS is due to endocarditis, carcinoid syndrome, or rheumatic heart disease.

Clinical Presentation

Patients with PS are often asymptomatic. Survival into adulthood is relatively common, even in the absence of surgical correction or valvotomy. Indeed, patients may reach their fourth to sixth decades of life without becoming cognizant of any symptoms or evidence of right-sided heart failure, even though significant pressure gradients may exist across the pulmonic valve. If right-sided heart failure does develop, particularly with age, patients may note fatigue, abdominal discomfort, abdominal swelling, or peripheral edema. Patients rarely present with chest pain or exertional syncope.

Findings on physical examination depend upon the severity of obstruction and the degree of myocardial compensation. The findings in many patients with PS may be subtle, due to the fact that most patients present with mild to moderate forms of the condition. Typically, PS is associated with a mid-systolic crescendo-decrescendo murmur heard best at the left sternal border. An ejection click may also be present, which usually decreases with inspiration. P2 is soft and delayed, producing a widely split S2, but one that will narrow with appropriate physiologic changes. Periodically, a right-sided S2 is appreciated at the left sternal border. A right ventricular lift may also be present. In patients with right ventricular failure, hepatomegaly, abdominal swelling, peripheral edema, and jugular venous distention with a prominent *a* wave may also be present.

Diagnosis and Management

TTE is the preferred test for diagnosing PS. TTE also provides information on the morphology of the leaflets, the severity of the stenosis, and any hemodynamic consequences associated with the pulmonic valve stenosis including right ventricular hypertrophy, right atrial enlargement, post-stenotic dilatation of the main pulmonary artery, and decreased right ventricular function. Typically, echocardiography will show thickened leaflets with reduced systolic excursion causing a domed appearance of the valve leaflets during ventricular contraction. In patients with severe PS, the domed appearance of the valve may appear during atrial contraction if the right ventricle has decreased compliance. Less commonly, a truly dysplastic pulmonic valve is visualized. Dysplastic valves are characterized by severely thickened and immobile leaflets. It is important to distinguish patients with truly dysplastic pulmonic valves as these patients are often not good candidates for percutaneous intervention. Transesophageal echocardiography (TEE) is not routinely used to evaluate PS, but may be used if TTE fails to provide adequate information regarding the diagnosis.

Adult patients with only mild PS generally do not require any intervention. In patients with mild to moderate PS, the ECG is frequently normal. In cases of severe PS, the ECG may show evidence of right-axis deviation, right atrial enlargement, and right ventricular hypertrophy. Right bundle branch block can also be seen in some patients with severe PS. Chest x-ray may show evidence of a post-stenotic dilated main pulmonary artery and reduced peripheral pulmonary vasculature markings.

Right heart catheterization is generally done only as a prelude to intervention. Simultaneous PA and RV pressures were obtained in this patient as shown in Figure 8.1.

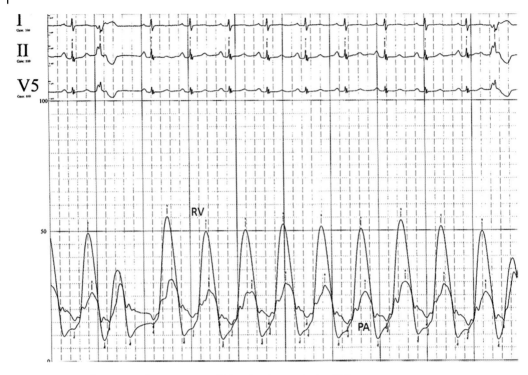

Figure 8.1 Simultaneous pulmonary artery (PA) and right ventricular (RV) pressures.

Further Reading

Goins, A., Tate, D.A., and Stouffer, G.A. (2018). Tricuspid and pulmonic valve disease. In: Netter Cardiology, 3e (ed. G. Stouffer, M.S. Runge, C. Patterson and J. Rossi), 336–340. Philadelphia PA. Chapter 48: Elsevier.

McCrindle, B.W. and Kan, J.S. (1991). Long-term results after balloon pulmonary valvuloplasty. *Circulation* 83: 1915.

Snellen, H.A., Hartman, H., Buis-Liem, T.N. et al. (1968). Pulmonic stenosis. *Circulation* 38: 93.

Stout, K.K. et al. (2018 Aug 10). 2018 AHA/ ACC Guideline for the management of adults with congenital heart disease: a report of the American College of Cardiology/American Heart Association Task Force on Clinical Practice Guidelines. *Journal of the American College of Cardiology* pii: S0735-1097(18)36846-3. https://doi. org/10.1016/j.jacc.2018.08.1029.

Weyman, A.E., Hurwitz, R.A., Girod, D.A. et al. (1977). Cross-sectional echocardiographic visualization of the stenotic pulmonary valve. *Circulation* 56: 769.

Case 9: A 31-Year-Old Man with Palpitations and Dizziness

You get a stat page from the Emergency Department to see a 31-year-old man brought in by Rescue Squad with complaints of palpitations and dizziness. Past medical history is remarkable for atrioventricular (AV) canal defect repair at birth.

On examination, he is pale and diaphoretic. Systolic blood pressure is ~80 mmHg. The ECG is below (Figure 9.1).

What is the rhythm and how would you treat this patient?

Atrial Flutter with 1 : 1 Conduction

The ECG shows a regular, wide complex tachycardia at a rate of approximately 250–270 bpm. The differential diagnosis is limited and includes atrial flutter with 1 : 1 conduction, AV reciprocating tachycardia, and ventricular tachycardia/flutter. If you are evaluating a patient with a heart rate near 300 bpm, make sure that you are confident

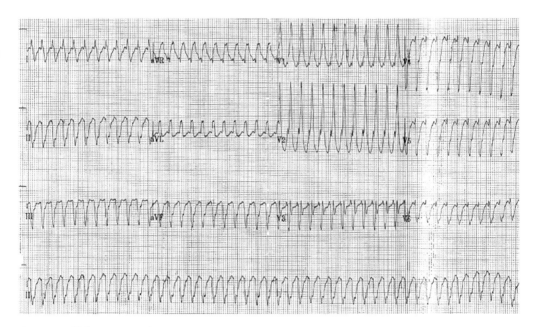

Figure 9.1 ECG on presentation.

Cardiology Board Review: ECG, Hemodynamic and Angiographic Unknowns, First Edition. Edited by George A. Stouffer.
© 2019 John Wiley & Sons Ltd. Published 2019 by John Wiley & Sons Ltd.

about the width of the QRS. Occasionally you will see a narrow complex rhythm at these rates, but ventricular rhythms are more common than supraventricular rhythms and occasionally a patient will be misdiagnosed because of a cursory review of an ECG.

If the patient is hemodynamically stable, you can attempt to make the diagnosis using carotid sinus massage or adenosine. If the patient is not tolerating the rate, immediate cardioversion is necessary.

This patient was given adenosine with the result as shown in Figure 9.2. 12-lead ECG after adenosine administration is shown in Figure 9.3.

Adenosine elicits transient AV block and enables the visualization of flutter waves (arrows). This patient had atrial flutter with one to one conduction. The patient underwent electrical cardioversion and the ECG after cardioversion is shown in Figure 9.3. Note the underlying RBBB (right bundle branch block) and LAFB (left anterior fascicular block) (remember that he had an AV canal defect repair). Long-term therapy would consist of an EP study with ablation of the bypass tract +/− medical treatment of atrial flutter (for rate control) if required.

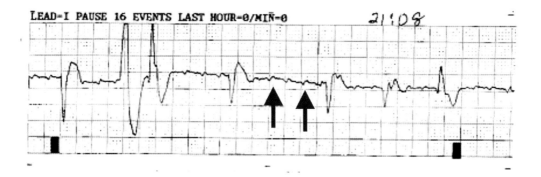

Figure 9.2 Rhythm strip during IV administration of adenosine.

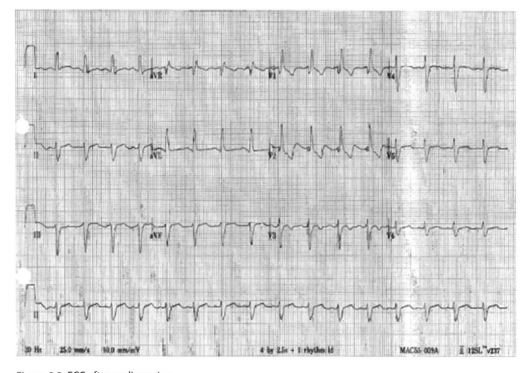

Figure 9.3 ECG after cardioversion.

Further Reading

Page, R.L., Joglar, J.A., Caldwell, M.A. et al. (2016). 2015 ACC/AHA/HRS guideline for the management of adult patients with supraventricular tachycardia: a report of the American College of Cardiology/American Heart Association Task Force on Clinical Practice Guidelines and the Heart Rhythm Society. *Journal of the American College of Cardiology* 67 (13): e27–e115. https://doi.org/10.1016/j.jacc.2015.08.856. Epub 2015 Sep 24.

Rahman, F., Wang, N., Yin, X. et al. (2016). Atrial flutter: clinical risk factors and adverse outcomes in the Framingham heart study. *Heart Rhythm* 13 (1): 233–240.

Case 10: An Unexpected Finding on a Coronary Angiogram

You are asked to see a 59-year-old female with exertional chest pain. An echocardiogram showed normal left ventricular function and no significant valvular abnormality. A nuclear exercise stress test was done which was remarkable for inferior wall ischemia. Your first picture with a right Judkins catheter is shown below (Figure 10.1). What is the interpretation?

Anomalous Circumflex Arising from the Right Coronary Artery

An anomalous circumflex is shown arising from the right coronary cusp near the ostium of the right coronary artery. This is confirmed during left coronary angiography when no circumflex is seen arising from the left main coronary artery (Figure 10.2).

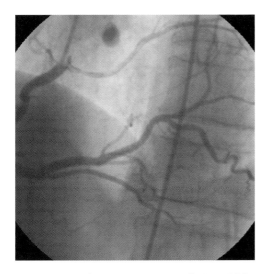

Figure 10.1 Right coronary angiography in an LAO (left anterior oblique) cranial view.

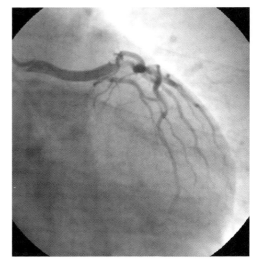

Figure 10.2 Left coronary angiography in an AP (anteroposterior) caudal view.

Cardiology Board Review: ECG, Hemodynamic and Angiographic Unknowns, First Edition. Edited by George A. Stouffer.
© 2019 John Wiley & Sons Ltd. Published 2019 by John Wiley & Sons Ltd.

Approximately 1–1.5% of patients undergoing coronary angiography will be found to have coronary anomalies. One of the most common variants is an anomalous left circumflex artery which is found in approximately 0.4–0.7% of patients. The circumflex anomaly arises from a separate ostium within the right sinus, or more rarely as a proximal branch of the right coronary artery. The arterial course of the circumflex relative to the aorta and pulmonary arteries can vary. While this anomaly is usually benign and asymptomatic, it has been reported to cause myocardial ischemia, sudden death, and myocardial infarction.

The patient had no epicardial disease to explain the nuclear stress test result. Lastly, note that this patient had a Class 2b indication for coronary angiography: CCS class 1 or 2 angina with demonstrable ischemia but no high-risk criteria on non-intensive testing.

Further Reading

Angelini, P., Velasco, J.A., and Flamm, S. (2002). Coronary anomalies: incidence, pathophysiology, and clinical relevance. *Circulation* 105: 2449–2454.

Cheezum, M.K., Ghoshhajra, B., Bittencourt, M.S. et al. (2016). Anomalous origin of the coronary artery arising from the opposite sinus: prevalence and outcomes in patients undergoing coronary CTA. *European Heart Journal Cardiovascular Imaging* 18 (2): 224–235.

Click, R.L., Holmes, D.R., Vlietstra, R.E. et al. (1989). Anomalous coronary arteries: location, degree of atherosclerosis and effect on survival – a report from the coronary artery surgery study. *Journal of the American College of Cardiology* 13 (3): 531–537.

Motta, P. and Santoro, J.E. (2017). Coronary artery anomalies. In: *Congenital Heart Disease in Pediatric and Adult Patients* (ed. A. Dabbagh, A.H. Conte and L. Lubin), 727–743. Cham: Springer.

Safak, O., Gursul, E., Yesil, M. et al. (2015). Prevalence of coronary artery anomalies in patients undergoing coronary artery angiography: a review of 16768 patients. A retrospective, single-center study. *Minerva Cardioangiologica* 63 (2): 113–120.

Case 11: A 26-Year-Old Man Who Collapses While Talking with Friends

You are asked to evaluate a 26-year-old man in the Emergency Department with syncope. He reports that he had sudden onset of light-headedness while talking with friends. He collapsed according to witnesses but had no seizure-like activity. He denies any preceding chest pain, nausea/vomiting, shortness of breath, or recent illness. He has had three prior episodes of syncope in the past – the first episode was four years ago followed by two episodes one year ago. On questioning, he also reports occasional palpitations associated with "not feeling well." What clues does the ECG provide in establishing a differential diagnosis (Figure 11.1)?

Arrhythmogenic Cardiomyopathy

This ECG should make you think of arrhythmogenic cardiomyopathy (AC; formerly known as arrhythmogenic ventricular dysplasia), especially in a young individual who presents with syncope. Important findings include T wave inversion in leads V1–V3 and a premature ventricular contraction (PVC) that originates from the right ventricle (note the left bundle branch block [LBBB] pattern by examining leads V1 and V5 on the rhythm strip).

AC is an inheritable heart disease caused by dysfunctional cardiac desmosomes, resulting

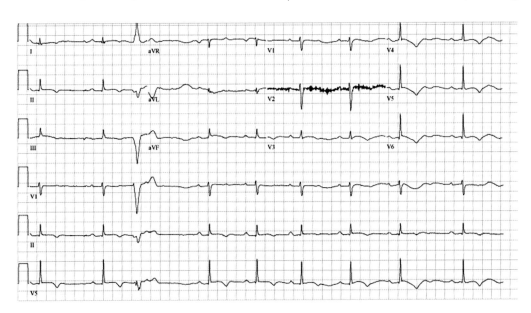

Figure 11.1 ECG on presentation.

Cardiology Board Review: ECG, Hemodynamic and Angiographic Unknowns, First Edition. Edited by George A. Stouffer.
© 2019 John Wiley & Sons Ltd. Published 2019 by John Wiley & Sons Ltd.

in patchy fibrofatty replacement and subsequent structural and functional alterations of the ventricles. Pathologically it is characterized by fibrofatty replacement of the right ventricular (RV) myocardium. In the early stage of the disease, structural changes are subtle and confined to a localized region of the RV, typically the inflow tract, outflow tract, or apex of the RV. Progression to more diffuse RV disease and left ventricular (LV) involvement, typically affecting the posterior lateral wall, is common. There is also a form of AC which predominantly affects the LV. The disease is genetically heterogeneous with mutations having been identified in multiple genes including desmoplakin, plakoglobin, plakophilin-2 (PKP2), desmoglein-2 (DSG2), desmocollin-2 (DSC2), transforming growth factor beta-3 (TGFß3), and TMEM43. The diagnosis of AC is based on the revised Task Force Criteria, which includes histological, ECG, arrhythmic, and genetic features of the disease as major and minor criteria.

The disease is characterized clinically by ventricular arrhythmias (originating from the RV) and/or RV pump failure. The prevalence is thought to be approximately 5 per 10 000, although the actual number may be higher because of difficulty in accurate diagnosis. The disease is progressive and as the myocardium is replaced by fibrofatty tissue the RV becomes dilated and dysfunctional. Individuals who come to medical attention are usually younger than 35 years and present with sudden death, chest pain, palpitations, fatigue, syncope, or rapid heart rate. Arrhythmias and sudden cardiac death are more common during exercise. In some series, AC is the second-most common cause of sudden cardiac death, after hypertrophic cardiomyopathy, in young individuals, and in at least one large series it was the most common cause of death in young athletes.

The gold standard for the diagnosis of AC is biopsy evidence of fibrofatty infiltration in the RV. This is not available in all patients and thus major and minor criteria for the diagnosis of AC have been established that include: (i) global or regional dysfunction and structural alterations; (ii) tissue characterization of wall; (iii) repolarization abnormalities; (iv) depolarization/conduction abnormalities; (v) arrhythmias; and (vi) family history. ECG changes listed under "Major diagnostic criteria" include: (i) inverted T waves in right precordial leads (V_1, V_2, and V_3) or beyond in individuals >14 years of age (in the absence of complete right bundle branch block QRS ≥120 ms); (ii) the presence of epsilon waves; small deflections at the terminal end of the QRS complex that are best seen in V1–V3 (Figure 11.2); and (iii) nonsustained or sustained ventricular tachycardia of left bundle branch morphology with superior axis (negative or indeterminate QRS in leads II, III, and aVF and positive in lead aVL). "Minor diagnostic criteria" include T wave inversion in the anterior precordial leads (V1–V2) in the absence of right bundle branch block (RBBB), ventricular tachycardia with a LBBB pattern (sustained or nonsustained; observed on ECG, Holter monitoring, or stress testing), or frequent PVCs (>500/24 hours). The amount of PVCs will often increase with exercise or emotional stress.

The differential diagnosis of these ECG findings includes myocarditis, Naxos Disease, sarcoid heart disease, dilated cardiomyopathy, or RV outflow tract tachycardia.

This patient was admitted to the hospital where telemetry showed multiple runs of nonsustained ventricular tachycardia. A transthoracic echocardiogram demonstrated normal LV function but a dilated right ventricle with decreased systolic function. A cardiac MRI was remarkable for fat interdigitation in the basilar RV free wall associated with diminished contractility at this site. During an electrophysiology study,

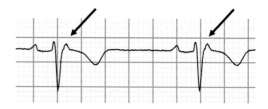

Figure 11.2 Epsilon waves.

monomorphic ventricular tachycardia with a left bundle branch morphology was induced and electronic voltage mapping was consistent with abnormal myocardium in the anterior free wall of the right ventricle. The patient was diagnosed with AC and treated with implantation of a cardioverter defibrillator.

Further Reading

Corrado, D., Wichter, T., Link, M.S. et al. (2015). Treatment of arrhythmogenic right ventricular cardiomyopathy/dysplasia: an international task force consensus statement. *European Heart Journal* 36: 3227–3237.

Haugaa, K.H., Basso, C., Badano, L.P. et al. (2017). Comprehensive multi-modality imaging approach in arrhythmogenic cardiomyopathy-an expert consensus document of the European Association of Cardiovascular Imaging. *European Heart Journal Cardiovascular Imaging* 18: 237–253.

Haugaa, K.H., Haland, T.F., Leren, I.S. et al. (2016). Arrhythmogenic right ventricular cardiomyopathy, clinical manifestations, and diagnosis. *Europace* 18: 965–972.

Marcus, F.I., McKenna, W.J., Sherrill, D. et al. (2010). Diagnosis of arrhythmogenic right ventricular cardiomyopathy/ dysplasia: proposed modification of the task force criteria. *Circulation* 121: 1533–1541.

Mazzanti, A., Ng, K., Faragli, A. et al. (2016). Arrhythmogenic right ventricular cardiomyopathy: clinical course and predictors of arrhythmic risk. *Journal of the American College of Cardiology* 68: 2540–2550.

Case 12: An Elderly Gentleman Who Passes Out While Working on His Farm

A 79-year-old man is referred to you for evaluation of exertional chest tightness and episodes of "passing out." He is otherwise healthy and takes no medications. He lives on a farm and has been very active throughout his whole life, and, until six months ago, he had been able to carry out duties on his farm without difficulty. During the last six months, he reports three episodes where he lost consciousness while working on his farm. Two of these episodes left him bruised but he has not broken any bones. He attributes these episodes to dehydration while working outside in the heat and humidity. He denies any associated bowel or bladder incontinence, or any preceding feelings of lightheadedness or nausea.

More recently, he reports onset of substernal tightness brought on with exertion. This usually occurs while carrying hay bales and using a shovel. The pain abates once he stops and rests for a few minutes.

Examination reveals a comfortable-appearing, elderly male with the following vital signs: BP = 133/73 mmHg, HR = 94 bpm, and O2 saturation of 98% on room air. Cardiovascular examination was remarkable for a regular rate and rhythm with a III/VI harsh, late-peaking, crescendo–decrescendo murmur heard best at the right upper sternal border with radiation to his carotids and obliteration of S2. An S4 gallop is auscultated. Carotid pulses are weak and appear to be slow-rising. ECG in the office shows normal sinus rhythm with evidence of left ventricular hypertrophy (LVH) (Figure 12.1). Complete blood count, metabolic panel, and thyroid function tests are within normal limits.

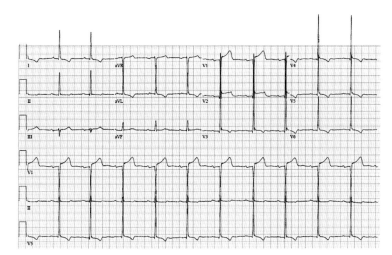

Figure 12.1 Electrocardiogram showing evidence of left ventricular hypertrophy (LVH). What is your diagnosis and what diagnostic test would you order?

Cardiology Board Review: ECG, Hemodynamic and Angiographic Unknowns, First Edition. Edited by George A. Stouffer.
© 2019 John Wiley & Sons Ltd. Published 2019 by John Wiley & Sons Ltd.

Aortic Stenosis

The presentation and physical examination are consistent with critical aortic stenosis (AS). A transthoracic echocardiogram was performed and confirmed a thick, heavily calcified aortic valve with severely reduced excursion of aortic leaflets as well as LVH. Flow studies across the aortic valve demonstrate an estimated valve area of $0.6\,cm^2$ consistent with a diagnosis of critical AS (Figure 12.2).

Valvular AS is typically caused by either calcification of a congenitally malformed valve, calcification of a normal trileaflet valve, or rheumatic heart disease (Otto and Prendergast 2014). This patient's constellation of symptoms, physical exam findings, and clinical tests are representative of senile calcific AS. His gradual reduction in exertional capacity, as well as syncope, are common signs of progressive AS. Many well-compensated patients may remain largely asymptomatic until the obstruction becomes severe. The presence of LVH on ECG and echocardiography is secondary to chronically elevated afterload as the heart compensates to reduce wall stress. Medications can be used to treat symptoms of fluid overload but no medication changes the natural history of AS. The cornerstone of management is centered on valve replacement using either a surgical or percutaneous approach.

Clinical Presentation

AS is a progressive disease characterized by a fixed left ventricular outflow obstruction which results in an inability to augment cardiac output to meet metabolic requirements (Otto and Prendergast 2014). This, in turn, leads to decreased exercise capacity, heart failure, and death from cardiovascular causes. Typically, symptoms of AS present between the ages of 50–70 years old in individuals with a congenitally malformed bicuspid aortic valve and after the age of 70 years in those with a normal trileaflet valve. The three cardinal symptoms of AS are syncope, angina, and dyspnea from heart failure.

Syncope is classically associated with exertion as there is an inability for cardiac output to increase because of aortic valve obstruction thus limiting the ability of the heart to provide adequate cerebral blood flow. Angina occurs when myocardial oxygen demand is exceeded by myocardial oxygen supply. As stated previously, elevation in afterload leads to LVH to compensate for increased wall stress which, in turn, leads to

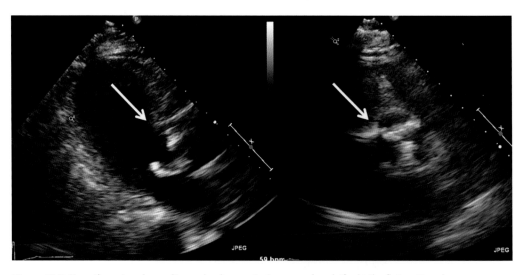

Figure 12.2 Transthoracic echocardiography demonstrates severely calcified trileaflet aortic valve.

an increase in myocardial oxygen consumption and demand (Gould and Carabello 2003). As left ventricular changes progress with increasing severity of AS and wall stress is not adequately normalized, patients may begin to experience angina, even in the absence of significant coronary artery disease (Gould and Carabello 2003). Additionally, LVH and chronic pressure overload of the LV results in worsening diastolic dysfunction due to diminished LV compliance. Over time, left atrial pressures also rise leading to left atrial dilation and transmission of increased pressures to the pulmonary venous circulation and capillary beds. Eventually, patients develop paroxysmal nocturnal dyspnea, orthopnea, dyspnea on exertion, and other signs of heart failure. Patients may also present with atrial fibrillation and findings of pulmonary hypertension due to chamber remodeling and chronic pressure overload.

Pathophysiology

Normal aortic valves are comprised of three cusps, each generally <1 mm thick with smooth contour (Dweck et al. 2012). Congenitally malformed valves are either unicuspid, bicuspid, tricuspid, or quadricuspid, with bicuspid valves being most common. Bicuspid aortic valves typically do not result in significant stenosis until later in adulthood.

Age-related senile calcific AS is the most common cause of AS in adults (Otto 2009). In calcific AS, the valve cusps become progressively thickened, fibrosed, and calcified leading to reduced cusp excursion and ultimately narrowing of the valve orifice (Otto 2009). Although the pathophysiology of calcific AS was traditionally thought to be secondary to wear-and-tear, research suggests multiple contributing factors: mechanical stress and endothelial damage, inflammation, angiogenesis, and proliferation and fibrosis (Dweck et al. 2012). In addition to the accumulation of fibrous tissue and

cellular remodeling, neurohormonal-mediated processes are thought to play a key role in the fibrotic process (Dweck et al. 2012). Although the rate of progression is variable, it appears to be more rapid in those patients with older age, renal insufficiency, hypertension, hyperlipidemia, and tobacco use.

Rheumatic AS is less common in the United States but remains a concern in third-world countries. Rheumatic AS is distinguished by the presence of commissural fusion and stiffening of the aortic cusps and is frequently associated with concomitant aortic regurgitation.

Diagnosis

Characterization of the severity of AS requires an integration of information regarding patient symptoms and clinical presentation, hemodynamics, valve anatomy, and left ventricular response to pressure overload (Otto 2009). On physical exam, AS is most classically recognized by a crescendo–decrescendo murmur heard best at the right upper sternal border that begins shortly after S1 with intensity highest during mid-to-late systole. In patients with LVH, a prominent S4 may be auscultated, representative of forceful atrial contraction against a stiff, noncompliant ventricle. As severity of AS evolves, the aortic component of S2 (A2) may become diminished or absent. A systolic thrill can sometimes be palpated with the patient sitting up and leaning forward. Evaluation of the carotid pulses may reveal a slow-rising, late-peaking, low amplitude pulse (*pulsus parvus et tardus)*. Laboratory evaluation should include evaluation of serum electrolyte levels, cardiac biomarkers, and B-type natriuretic peptide (BNP). Electrocardiography would likely show findings associated with LVH and sometimes also left atrial enlargement.

Echocardiographic evaluation includes assessment of valve anatomy, LV function and size, aortic root size, maximum transvalvular velocity, and mean and peak gradients

Table 12.1 Quantification of AS severity based on echocardiographic measurements as delineated in the 2014 AHA/ACC Guidelines for the Management of Patients with Valvular Heart Disease.

	Mild	Moderate	Severe
Aortic jet velocity (m/s)	2.6–2.9	3.0–4.0	>4.0
Mean gradient (mmHg)	<20	20–40	>40
AVA (cm^2)	>1.5	1.0–1.5	<1.0
Indexed AVA (cm^2/m^2)	>0.85	0.60–0.85	<0.6

which are fundamental features of current AHA/ACC guidelines on management of severe AS (Table 12.1) (Nishimura et al. 2014). Severe AS is defined as a peak aortic valve velocity of >4.0 m/s and a corresponding mean transvalvular gradient >40 mmHg (in the presence of normal cardiac output) as well as aortic valve area (AVA) of <1.0 cm^2 (normal 3.0–4.0 cm^2). Typically, an AVA of 1.5–2.0 cm^2 is considered mild AS and an AVA of 1.0–1.5 cm^2 is considered moderate AS. In patients with reduced LV systolic function and low stroke volume index (<34 ml/m^2), dobutamine stress echocardiography can be performed to better evaluate hemodynamic severity of the AS (Nishimura et al. 2014). In patients with severe AS who receive escalating doses of dobutamine, the transvalvular stroke volume, velocity, and gradient rise markedly with an unchanged aortic valve area. CT and MR imaging can be helpful to gauge extent of valvular calcification as well as better comprehend LV volume, function, and mass. Additionally, invasive hemodynamic assessment of AS with cardiac catheterization can be invaluable, particularly in circumstances where echocardiographic and clinical assessments are conflicting.

Management

Currently, there are no medical therapies available to prevent or slow progression of AS. The only definitive treatment in adults is aortic valve replacement (AVR) which can be performed either via a surgical or percutaneous approach. The latent period for progression in AS before symptoms develop can be as long as 10–15 years (Otto 2009). Once symptoms become apparent, prognosis is poor unless appropriate treatment is provided. Indeed, the classical doctrine regarding prognosis suggests time from symptoms to mortality to be five years in patients presenting with angina, three years in patients presenting with syncope, and two years in those presenting with heart failure. As such, it is critical to follow patients closely as appropriate timing of symptom recognition has significant clinical implications. Annual surveillance echocardiography should be performed in patients with severe AS to evaluate for worsening LVH and hemodynamics. Exercise testing should be performed with caution in patients who report being asymptomatic but high clinical index of suspicion for reduced exertional capacity is present. Surgical AVR has long been the standard of care for management of patients with severe AS, but a growing number of patients are receiving treatment with transcutaneous aortic valve replacement (TAVR).

AVR is indicated for symptomatic patients with severe, high-gradient AS (class 1), asymptomatic patients with severe AS and reduced LVEF <50% (class 1), and in those patients with severe AS who are undergoing a concomitant cardiac surgery (class 1) (Nishimura et al. 2014). AVR is reasonable in asymptomatic patients with very severe AS – peak velocity >5.0 m/s (class 2a) or with severe AS and decreased exercise tolerance or reduction in BP with exercise (class 2a) (Nishimura et al. 2014). AVR is also reasonable in symptomatic patients with severe AS with low-flow/low-gradient AS in whom a dobutamine stress test reveals transvalvular velocity >4.0 m/s or mean gradient >40 mmHg and an estimated AVA < 1.0 cm^2 (class 2a) (Nishimura et al. 2014). AVR is reasonable in symptomatic patients with low-flow/low-gradient severe AS with LVEF >50% if clinical, hemodynamic, and anatomic data support valve obstruction as the most likely cause of symptoms (2a) (Nishimura et al. 2014). Finally, AVR is reasonable to perform in patients with moderate AS who are undergoing a concomitant cardiac surgery (class 2a) (Nishimura et al., 2014). Typically, balloon aortic valvuloplasty (BAV) is not recommended due to lack of proven durability. However, in very select cases, BAV may be reasonable as a bridge to surgery in unstable patients or as a palliative measure.

References

Dweck, M.R., Boon, N.A., and Newby, D.E. (2012). Calcific aortic stenosis: A disease of the valve and the Myocardium. *Journal of the American College of Cardiology* 60 (19): 1854–1863.

Gould, K.L. and Carabello, B.A. (2003). Why angina in aortic stenosis with Normal coronary arteriograms? *Circulation* 107 (25): 3121–3123.

Nishimura, R.A., Otto, C.M., Bonow, R.O. et al. (2014). AHA/ACC guideline for the management of patients with valvular heart disease: a report of the American College of Cardiology/American Heart Association Task Force on Practice Guidelines. *The Journal of Thoracic and Cardiovascular Surgery* 148 (1): e1–e132.

Otto, C.M. (2009). Calcific aortic valve disease: outflow obstruction is the end stage of a systemic disease process. *European Heart Journal* 30 (16): 1940–1942.

Otto, C.M. and Prendergast, B. (2014). Aortic Valve Stenosis – From Risk to Severe Valve Obstruction. *The New England Journal of Medicine* 371 (8): 744–756.

Case 13: A 46-Year-Old Woman with Dyspnea on Exertion and Daily Emesis

You are asked to see a 46-year-old female in your clinic for evaluation of two weeks of accelerating dyspnea on exertion and daily emesis. She reported some global fatigue and being "short-winded" over the last two to three months. She initially attributed these symptoms to her hectic schedule but over the last two weeks her dyspnea progressed, becoming so severe that walking several steps in her house is completely exhausting. She also reports episodes where she feels as though she may pass out but denies frank syncope. What is the rhythm on the ECG below (Figure 13.1)?

Ectopic Atrial Rhythm

The sinoatrial (SA) node, the normal pacemaker of the heart, is located in the posterior part of the right atrium at the junction of the superior vena cava. In normal sinus rhythm, the p wave axis (determined from the limb leads) varies from 0 to +75 (i.e. directed inferiorly and leftward). The P wave is always upright in leads I and II. In an ectopic atrial rhythm, the P wave axis is generally abnormal and P waves are negative in either lead I or lead II. The morphology of the P wave and the direction of the frontal plane P wave axis

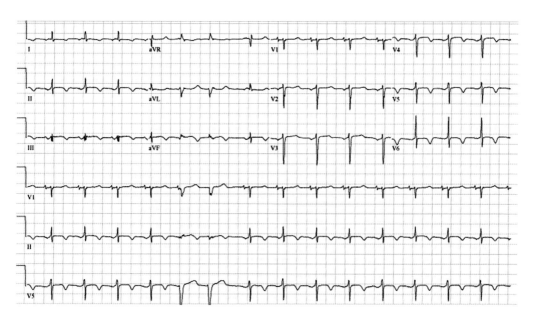

Figure 13.1 ECG on presentation.

Cardiology Board Review: ECG, Hemodynamic and Angiographic Unknowns, First Edition. Edited by George A. Stouffer.
© 2019 John Wiley & Sons Ltd. Published 2019 by John Wiley & Sons Ltd.

depends on the location of the automatic focus and the pathway of atrial activation. For example, when the focus is lower in the atrium, the P wave in the inferior leads is inverted. In general, in ectopic atrial rhythm the rate <100 bpm and the PR interval is normal. If the P wave morphology varies and there are multiple P wave morphologies, think of wandering atrial pacemaker.

Ectopic atrial rhythm is generally a disorder of increased automaticity, although reentry mechanisms can also be a cause. Increased automaticity can be observed in tissue within the atria, the AV junction, or the vena cava or pulmonary veins. Enhanced automaticity results from increased diastolic phase 4 depolarization causing an increase in rate of activation. If the rate of the ectopic focus exceeds that of the sinus node, then the ectopic focus will become the predominant pacemaker of the heart.

The patient undergoes an echocardiogram and an apical 4 chamber view is shown in Figure 13.2. What is the diagnosis?

Atrial Myxoma

This patient was found on echocardiography to have an atrial myxoma (Figure 13.2). There are no ECG findings diagnostic of a myxoma.

Rather the ECG findings associated with a myxoma are indirect and depend on the location of the tumor. If the tumor is only in the atria, there can be P wave abnormalities or atrial arrhythmias (including ectopic atrial rhythm as in this patient) on ECG. If the tumor extends into the mitral annulus, and affects the function of the valve, findings associated with mitral valve disease, such as atrial enlargement, can also be found on the ECG. Right bundle branch block and ST abnormalities have been reported with myxomas. Lastly, diffuse T wave inversion and/or ventricular ectopy (note the fifth and sixth beats), as seen on this ECG, can also be present.

Myxomas are the most common type of cardiac tumors in all age groups accounting for approximately three-quarters of cardiac tumors treated surgically. Most myxomas arise from the atrial septum. They occur more commonly in the left atrium (75–90%) than in the right atrium. Myxomas can also be biatrial with the most common arrangement being attachment of two stalks to the opposite side of the same area of the septum. Right atrial myxomas tend to be more sessile than left atrial myxomas, with a wider attachment to the atrial septum. Right atrial tumors are equally likely to be myxomas and sarcomas. Myxomas can be polypoid, round, or oval and are gelati-

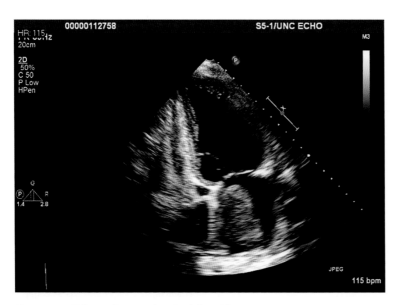

Figure 13.2 Echocardiogram showing left atrial mass.

nous. They can have have a smooth or lobulated surface and are usually white, yellow, or brown in color. Symptoms from myxomas can be due to systemic emboli or mechanical interference with cardiac function.

Although atrial myxomas are typically benign, local recurrence due to inadequate resection or malignant change has been reported.

Further Reading

Abu Abeeleh, M., Saleh, S., Alhaddad, E. et al. (2017). Cardiac myxoma: clinical characteristics, surgical intervention, intra-operative challenges and outcome. *Perfusion* 32 (8): 686–690.

Rahman, S.M., Kibria, M.G., Rahim, A.A. et al. (2015). Clinical presentation of left atrial Myxoma in relation to anatomic and pathologic type. *Cardiovascular Journal* 8 (1): 19–22.

Vroomen, M., Houthuizen, P., Khamooshian, A. et al. (2015). Long-term follow-up of 82 patients after surgical excision of atrial myxomas. *Interactive Cardiovascular and Thoracic Surgery* 21 (2): 183–188.

Case 14: A Pregnant Woman with Palpitations

A 34-year-old female who is 26 weeks pregnant is referred to you by her obstetrician for evaluation of "palpitations." This is her first pregnancy and she has no significant past medical history. She notes a history of palpitations as a teenager, but she was not evaluated at that time because her symptoms spontaneously resolved. Her current episodes began early in her pregnancy and now occur sporadically several times a week, usually when she is exerting herself. She does not have associated chest discomfort or shortness of breath. She has not had any syncope, but she feels lightheaded if standing when episodes occur. Aside from palpitations, her pregnancy has been otherwise uneventful.

Examination shows a comfortable-appearing, gravid female with blood pressure of 134/68 mmHg, heart rate of 82 bpm, and O_2 saturation of 97% on room air. Cardiovascular examination is normal. Radial and dorsalis pedis pulses are normal. 1+ pitting pedal edema is present bilaterally. Lungs are clear.

ECG in the office is completely normal. Complete blood count (CBC), metabolic panel, thyroid function are normal. Urine toxicology is negative.

An echocardiogram is scheduled for the following week, and a cardiac event monitor is ordered. However, prior to obtaining these studies, the patient presents to the local Emergency Department with palpitations and dizziness. The following ECG is obtained (Figure 14.1).

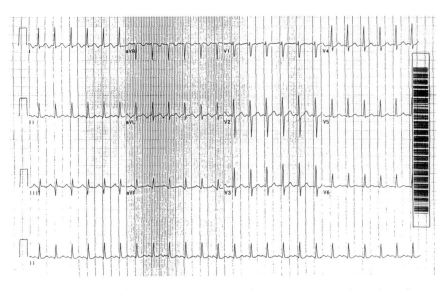

Figure 14.1 ECG tracing from the emergency room showing narrow complex tachycardia.

Cardiology Board Review: ECG, Hemodynamic and Angiographic Unknowns, First Edition. Edited by George A. Stouffer.
© 2019 John Wiley & Sons Ltd. Published 2019 by John Wiley & Sons Ltd.

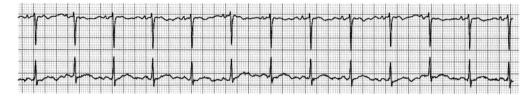

Figure 14.2 Telemetry showing normal sinus rhythm after adenosine.

In the Emergency Department she is given intravenous adenosine with resolution of the tachycardia (Figure 14.2). What is the diagnosis?

Focal Atrial Tachycardia

This 34-year old pregnant female presents with symptomatic narrow complex tachycardia with a ventricular rate of 160 bpm. The QRS axis is normal. The RP interval is longer than the PR interval during tachycardia. The differential diagnosis for "long RP tachycardia" includes sinus tachycardia, atrial tachycardia (AT), atrial flutter, atypical AV nodal reentrant tachycardia (AVNRT), and orthodromic AV reciprocating tachycardia (AVRT). The P waves during tachycardia in leads II, III, aVF are inverted (Figure 14.1) and clearly different from the sinus P waves seen after adenosine (Figure 14.2). Atrial flutter may present with similar ECG features but would not be expected to reliably terminate with adenosine. This patient had AT.

Clinical Presentation

Focal AT can be sustained or nonsustained and is usually at an atrial rate of 100–250 bpm. Sustained focal AT is a relatively uncommon form of supraventricular tachycardia (SVT), diagnosed in approximately 5–15% of patients referred for electrophysiology study and in 3–17% of the patients referred for SVT ablation (Page et al. 2016). The preva-

lence of AT increases with age and in those with structural heart disease and lung disease (Porter et al. 2004).

Nonsustained focal AT is common and often does not require treatment. Nonsustained AT can however be associated with symptoms similar to other forms of SVT with palpitations, dizziness, and pre-syncope sometimes associated with chest discomfort and dyspnea. Incessant AT is unusual but can result in tachycardia-induced cardiomyopathy (Medi et al. 2009). Paroxysmal AT is often seen in hospitalized patients who are acutely ill or those undergoing surgery in which increased adrenergic drive and catecholamine excess can precipitate arrhythmia.

Pathophysiology

Focal atrial activation can be either caused by automaticity, triggered activity, or microreentry although determination of the exact mechanism for any particular AT is difficult and unlikely to affect ongoing management (Page et al. 2016). In general, focal AT most often arises from a single area of atrial activation which spreads centrifugally, although in some patients, two or more unique foci are present. Focal AT has been localized to the crista terminalis, right or left atrial free wall or appendage, tricuspid or mitral annulus, paraseptal or paranodal areas, pulmonary veins, coronary sinus, and coronary cusps, but it originates more frequently from the right atrium than from the left atrium. Most focal AT arises from the right atrium, often along the long axis of the crista terminalis

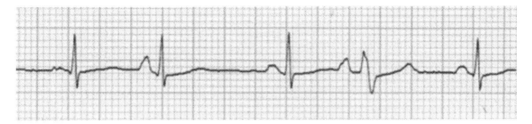

Figure 14.3 An example of multifocal atrial tachycardia (MAT). Notice the varying P wave morphologies.

(Kalman et al. 1998). Left atrial AT most often originates from the ostia of the pulmonary veins. Left atrial AT may be associated with atrial fibrillation (AF) in patients who are at risk for AF due to other conditions, however, AT in itself is not a risk factor for future development of AF.

When multiple foci result in at least three different P wave morphologies on ECG, the term multifocal atrial tachycardia (MAT) is employed (Figure 14.3). MAT is particularly prevalent in older males with lung disease. Typical atrial flutter is distinct from focal AT in that it is caused by macroreentry, characterized by a larger circuit resulting in atrial activation over the entire atrial cycle length, i.e. no isoelectric baseline on ECG (Anselme 2008).

Diagnosis

AT on ECG appears as a regular, narrow complex tachycardia with an atrial rate of 100–250 bpm. The RP interval is typically "long" (i.e. RP interval > PR interval). The differential diagnosis for long RP tachycardia additionally includes sinus tachycardia, AT, atrial flutter, atypical AVNRT, and orthodromic AVRT. P waves in AT are typically distinct from sinus P waves and comparison to a prior ECG in normal sinus rhythm may aid in the diagnosis. An exception to this is perinodal AT or sinus node reentrant tachycardia in which P waves appear identical in sinus rhythm and during tachyarrhythmia (Page et al. 2016). The atrial to ventricular relationship in AT is typically 1 : 1, however,

the presence of AV block during tachycardia is highly suggestive of AT versus AVRT or AVNRT.

Localization of Focus of AT

P wave morphology can be used to estimate the origin of the AT. Positive P waves in lead I and aVL with biphasic or negative P waves in V1 suggest a right atrial focus. AT from the pulmonary veins results in entirely positive P waves in lead V1 and often all precordial leads, and isoelectric or negative P waves in lead aVL. Left PV foci result in isoelectric or negative P waves in lead I whereas right PV foci result in positive P waves in lead I. In general, a positive P wave in lead V1 and negative P waves in leads I and aVL are correlated to ATs arising from the left atrium. Positive P waves in leads II, III, and aVF suggest that the origin of AT is from the cranial portion of either atria. Shorter P wave duration is correlated to AT arising from the paraseptal tissue versus the right or left atrial free wall. The precise location of the focal AT is ultimately confirmed by mapping during EP studies.

Management

In the acute setting, AT in the hemodynamically stable patient can be treated with intravenous adenosine, beta blocker, or calcium channel blocker. IV amiodarone may also be effective in slowing the ventricular rate. Adenosine may be used if the diagnosis of AT is unclear. Observing persistent AT despite adenosine-induced transient AV block makes AVRT or AVNRT less likely. Adenosine is often effective in terminating AT due to triggered activity but not due to reentry or automaticity. Hemodynamically unstable patients should receive synchronized cardioversion. For long-term management, patients with symptomatic AT should be considered for electrophysiology study and catheter ablation as an alternative to pharmacological therapy. Oral beta blockers and calcium channel blockers can be used prior to catheter ablation or in patients who do not wish to undergo ablation. Patients with newly diagnosed AT should receive echocardiography to evaluate for structural heart disease.

Sinus Node Reentrant Tachycardia

Sinus node reentrant tachycardia is an uncommon type of focal AT and is generally associated with paroxysmal episodes of tachycardia at rates of 100–150 bpm. It arises from a microreentrant circuit in the region of the sinoatrial node and thus P wave morphology is identical to that of sinus tachycardia. Abrupt onset and termination and a longer RP interval than that observed during normal sinus rhythm are characteristics that distinguish sinus node reentry from sinus tachycardia.

References

Anselme, F. (2008). Macroreentrant atrial tachycardia: pathophysiological concepts. *Heart Rhythm* 5 (6 Suppl): S18–S21. https://doi.org/10.1016/j.hrthm.2008.01.034. Epub 2008 Jan 29.

Kalman, J.M., Olgin, J.E., Karch, M.R. et al. (1998). "Cristal tachycardias": origin of right atrial tachycardias from the crista terminalis identified by intracardiac echocardiography. *Journal of the American College of Cardiology* 31 (2): 451–459.

Medi, C., Kalman, J.M., Haqqani, H. et al. (2009). Tachycardia-mediated cardiomyopathy secondary to focal atrial tachycardia: long-term outcome after catheter ablation. *Journal of the American College of Cardiology* 53 (19): 1791–1797. https://doi.org/10.1016/j.jacc.2009.02.014.

Page, R.L., Joglar, J.A., Caldwell, M.A. et al. (2016). 2015 ACC/AHA/HRS Guideline for the Management of Adult Patients With Supraventricular Tachycardia: A Report of the American College of Cardiology/American Heart Association Task Force on Clinical Practice Guidelines and the Heart Rhythm Society. *Journal of the American College of Cardiology* 67 (13): e27–e115. https://doi.org/10.1016/j.jacc.2015.08.856. Epub 2015 Sep 24.

Porter, M.J., Morton, J.B., Denman, R. et al. (2004). Influence of age and gender on the mechanism of supraventricular tachycardia. *Heart Rhythm* 1 (4): 393–396. https://doi.org/10.1016/j.hrthm.2004.05.007.

Case 15: Is this a Positive Brockenbrough Sign?

You are performing a left heart catheterization on a 58-year-old male with a loud systolic murmur heard throughout the precordium. Measuring simultaneous pressures in the left ventricle and aorta you obtain the following pressure tracing (Figure 15.1). What is the diagnosis?

Hypertrophic Obstructive Cardiomyopathy with a Brockenbrough Sign

The Brockenbrough–Braunwald–Morrow sign (more commonly known as the Brockenbrough sign) was originally described in 1961. This sign

is present if the aortic pulse pressure falls in the first normal beat post-PVC (Figure 15.2). While originally thought to be specific for hypertrophic obstructive cardiomyopathy (HOCM), it has since been described in some cases of aortic stenosis.

Outflow tract obstruction in patients with HOCM is "dynamic," which means the resistance to flow changes depending on filling pressures, afterload (e.g. aortic pressure), and force of contractility. The obstruction of the left ventricular outflow tract (LVOT) changes in severity depending on the force of systolic contraction and the dimensions of the left ventricular (LV; in contrast to aortic stenosis which is a fixed obstruction since it is valvular and not muscular). In HOCM,

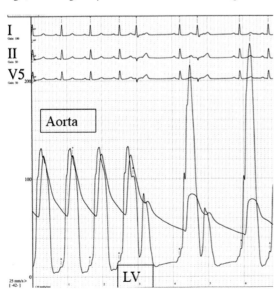

Figure 15.1 Simultaneous left ventricular (LV) and aortic pressures.

Cardiology Board Review: ECG, Hemodynamic and Angiographic Unknowns, First Edition. Edited by George A. Stouffer.
© 2019 John Wiley & Sons Ltd. Published 2019 by John Wiley & Sons Ltd.

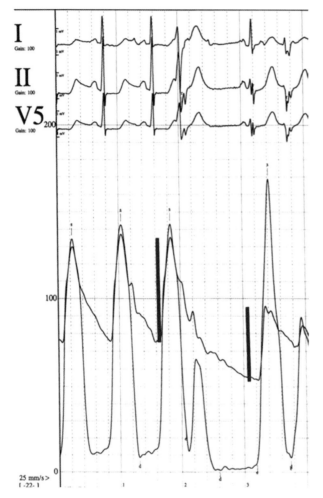

Figure 15.2 Simultaneous left ventricular (LV) and aortic pressures. The red lines indicate pulse pressure before and after a PVC.

LVOT gradients can be provoked using methods that decrease filling pressures and stroke volume (e.g. Valsalva maneuver or nitroglycerin) or methods that increase the force of contraction (post-PVC or isoproterenol infusion).

On physical examination, there is often a harsh crescendo–decrescendo systolic murmur that begins slightly after S1, is heard best at the left sternal border, and may radiate to the base of the heart. If significant mitral regurgitation is present, there may also be a holosystolic murmur heard at the apex that radiates to the axilla. If the mitral regurgita-tion is due to systolic anterior motion of the mitral valve, there may be a posteriorly directed jet, producing a mid to late systolic murmur at the apex.

Differentiating a systolic murmur related to LVOT obstruction from aortic stenosis can be done using a series of maneuvers and position changes. An increase in the intensity of an LVOT obstructive murmur will be heard with maneuvers that decrease preload (e.g. standing up or during a Valsalva maneuver). A decrease in intensity is heard when going from a standing to sitting position, with hand-grip, or following passive elevation of the legs.

Further Reading

Braunwald, E., Lambrew, C.T., Morrow, A.G. et al. (1964). Idiopathic hypertrophic subaortic stenosis. *Circulation* 30 (Suppl IV): IV–1.

Brockenbrough, E.C., Braunwald, E., and Morrow, A.G. (1961). A hemodynamic technique for the detection of hypertrophic subaortic stenosis. *Circulation*. 23: 189–194.

Gersh, B.J., Maron, B.J., Bonow, R.O. et al. (2011). 2011 ACCF/AHA guideline for the diagnosis and treatment of hypertrophic cardiomyopathy: Executive summary: A report of the American College of Cardiology Foundation/American Heart Association Task Force on Practice Guidelines. *Journal of the American College of Cardiology*. 58: 2703–2738.

Case 16: Dyspnea in a Woman Who Is Five Months Postpartum

You are asked to see a 19-year-old female, 5 months postpartum, with a prior history of myocarditis who presented to the Emergency Department with chest pain and shortness of breath. These symptoms were preceded by a "few days" of fever and cough. She also describes an episode where she felt dizzy and like she was going to pass out. On physical examination, her blood pressure is 98/46 mm Hg and her heart rate is 60 bpm. Her cardiovascular exam is normal. An ECG (electrocardiogram) is shown below (Figure 16.1). What is the diagnosis?

Complete Heart Block

This ECG shows complete heart block (CHB) which is also known as third-degree heart block. The ECG is notable for complete dissociation of the P waves and QRS complexes as the atria and ventricles are electrically independent of each other. The atrial rate is approximately 130 bpm while the ventricular rate is 61 bpm. The atrial rate is calculated by measuring the PP interval (note that the P wave can be hidden within the QRS or T waves). A clue to CHB is the presence of vari-

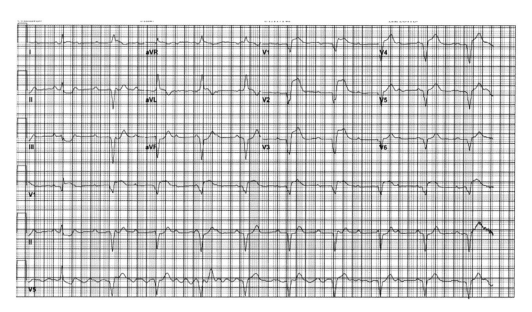

Figure 16.1 ECG on presentation.

Cardiology Board Review: ECG, Hemodynamic and Angiographic Unknowns, First Edition. Edited by George A. Stouffer.
© 2019 John Wiley & Sons Ltd. Published 2019 by John Wiley & Sons Ltd.

able and random PR intervals. In this case the PR intervals are different in nearly every beat, thus highlighting the independence of the atria and ventricles.

The atrial rate is generally determined by the sinus node although CHB can also occur with atrial arrhythmias.

In an individual with CHB, the ventricular rate is determined by an escape rhythm which can vary from 20 to 70 bpm. In general, the lower in the conduction system that the escape pacemaker originates from, the wider the QRS complex and the slower the rate will be. The escape rhythm in this case is probably within the AV (atrioventricular) node or His bundle as the QRS is not excessively wide.

Criteria for diagnosing CHB include: (i) regular P waves at a rate faster than the ventricular rate; (ii) regular QRS complexes at a rate slower than the P waves; and (iii) no relationship between the P waves and QRS complexes with variable and random PR intervals.

Be careful not to confuse CHB with AV dissociation from other causes. For example, in accelerated idioventricular rhythm, a pacemaker focus originates from within the ventricles at the rate that is greater than the atrial rate. This results in AV dissociation but does not imply impairment in conduction through the AV node; rather the atria and ventricles beat independently because the ventricles are going faster than the atria.

CHB in this age group can be congenital or acquired. Causes of acquired CHB include medications (e.g. digitalis preparations), Lyme disease, endocarditis, acute rheumatic fever, infiltrative diseases, or acute myocardial infarction.

Echocardiography in this patient showed severe left ventricular dysfunction and myocardial biopsies showed inflammation and necrosis consistent with acute myocarditis. A temporary pacemaker was placed. Following treatment, left ventricular function improved and the CHB resolved (Figure 16.2).

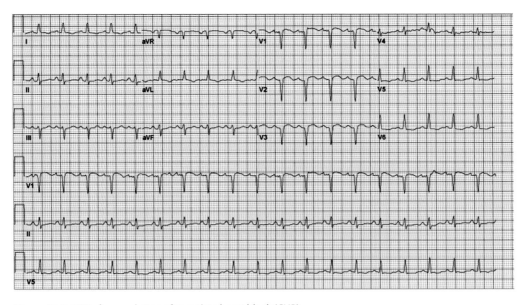

Figure 16.2 ECG after resolution of complete heart block (CHB).

Further Reading

Bordachar, P., Zachary, W., Ploux, S. et al. (2013). Pathophysiology, clinical course, and management of congenital complete atrioventricular block. *Heart Rhythm* 10 (5): 760–766.

Epstein, A.E., JP, D.M., Ellenbogen, K.A. et al. (2008). ACC/AHA/HRS 2008 guidelines for device-based therapy of cardiac rhythm abnormalities: a report of the American College of Cardiology/American Heart Association Task Force on Practice Guidelines (Writing Committee to Revise the ACC/AHA/NASPE 2002 Guideline Update for Implantation of Cardiac Pacemakers and Antiarrhythmia Devices) developed in collaboration with the American Association for Thoracic Surgery and Society of Thoracic Surgeons. *Journal of the American College of Cardiology* 51 (21): e1–e62.

Case 17: Can you Identify This Coronary Anomaly?

You are asked to see a 62-year-old female with exertional chest pain. An echocardiogram showed normal left ventricular function and no significant valvular abnormality. An exercise stress test was done during which the patient exercised for 10 minutes on a Bruce protocol with normal blood pressure and heart rate respond. She had 2 mm of ST depression at peak exercise and was referred for coronary angiography. Your first two pictures with a right Judkins catheter are shown in Figures 17.1 and 17.2. What is the interpretation?

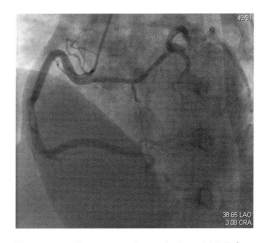

Figure 17.1 Coronary angiography in an LAO (left anterior oblique) view.

Single Coronary Artery Arising from the Right Coronary Cusp

In the normal heart, the right coronary artery (RCA) arises from the right coronary sinus and the left main coronary artery arises from the left coronary sinus. The RCA runs in the right atrioventricular (AV) groove. Marginal branch(s) usually arises from the mid RCA and supply the right ventricular wall. The distal RCA gives rise to right posterolateral branches and the posterior descending artery (PDA) in 85% of cases (defined as right dominance). The PDA arises from the left circumflex (LCx) in 8% of cases (defined as left dominance), and from both the RCA and LCx in 7% of cases (defined as codominance). The PDA runs in the posterior interventricular groove and supplies the posterior aspect of the interventricular septum.

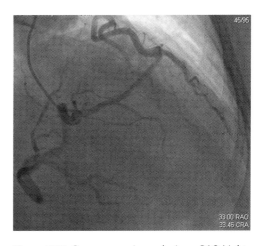

Figure 17.2 Coronary angiography in an RAO (right anterior oblique) cranial view.

Cardiology Board Review: ECG, Hemodynamic and Angiographic Unknowns, First Edition. Edited by George A. Stouffer.
© 2019 John Wiley & Sons Ltd. Published 2019 by John Wiley & Sons Ltd.

The left main coronary artery bifurcates into the left anterior descending (LAD) and LCx. In a minority of cases, the left main coronary artery trifurcates into the LAD, ramus intermedius artery, and LCx. The LAD runs in the anterior interventricular toward the apex of the heart and supplies the anterior wall of the left ventricle. Septal perforator branches arise from the LAD and supply the interventricular septum. Diagonal branches also arise from the LAD and supply the anterolateral wall of the left ventricle. The LCx runs in the left AV groove and gives off obtuse marginal branches that supply the posterolateral wall of the left ventricle. As noted above, in a minority of cases the PDA will arise from the LCx. The sinoatrial (SA) node artery arises from the RCA in approximately 70% of individuals and from the LCx in the remaining 30%. The origin of the SA node artery is not dependent on which artery is dominant. The AV node artery is generally the first and longest inferior septal perforating branch of the RCA (90%) or LCx (10%). The origin of the AV node artery is dependent on which artery is dominant.

Coronary artery anomalies are typically a result of abnormal embryologic development and are found in 1–1.5% of cases. Most coronary artery anomalies are clinically benign. The most common coronary artery anomaly is the presence of separate origins of the LAD and LCx, which occurs in 0.4–1% of cases and may be associated with a bicuspid aortic valve. Clinically significant anomalies include a coronary artery originating from the opposite coronary sinus (e.g. left main coronary artery originating from the right coronary sinus), the presence of a single coronary ostium leading to a single coronary artery, a coronary artery coursing between the great vessels (e.g. between the aorta and pulmonary artery), and a coronary artery leading to decreased oxygenation of myocardium (e.g. a coronary artery originating from the pulmonary artery or a coronary artery-ventricular fistula).

Single coronary artery arising from the aortic trunk via a single coronary ostium and providing for perfusion of the entire myocardium is rare with a prevalence of approximately 0.024–0.066% of patients undergoing coronary angiography. There are various classifications according to the site of origin and anatomical distribution of the branches. In general, cases are divided into "R" right-type and "L" left-type according to the site of origin of the single coronary artery from the right or left sinus of Valsalva and then subdivided depending on the anatomical course of the artery.

Lastly, note that this patient had a Class 2b indication for coronary angiography: CCS class 1 or 2 angina with demonstrable ischemia but no high-risk criteria on nonintensive testing.

Further Reading

Angelini, P., Velasco, J.A., and Flamm, S. (2002). Coronary anomalies: incidence, pathophysiology, and clinical relevance. *Circulation* 105: 2449–2454.

Cheezum, M.K., Ghoshhajra, B., Bittencourt, M.S. et al. (2016). Anomalous origin of the coronary artery arising from the opposite sinus: prevalence and outcomes in patients undergoing coronary CTA. *European Heart Journal Cardiovascular Imaging* 18 (2): 224–235.

Click, R.L., Holmes, D.R., Vlietstra, R.E. et al. (1989). Anomalous coronary arteries: location, degree of atherosclerosis and effect on survival – a report from the coronary artery surgery study. *Journal of the American College of Cardiology* 13 (3): 531–537.

Motta, P. and Santoro, J.E. (2017). Coronary artery anomalies. In: Congenital Heart Disease in Pediatric and Adult Patients (ed. A. Dabbagh, A.H. Conte and L. Lubin), 727–743. Cham: Springer.

Safak, O., Gursul, E., Yesil, M. et al. (2015). Prevalence of coronary artery anomalies in patients undergoing coronary artery angiography: a review of 16768 patients. A retrospective, single-center study. *Minerva Cardioangiologica* 63 (2): 113–120.

Case 18: Why Is this Patient Short of Breath?

A 50-year-old male is referred to you for evaluation of shortness of breath. Approximately three years ago, he began having complaints of dyspnea on exertion. The symptoms progressed until he was short of breath walking up one flight of stairs. Approximately one year ago, he began to notice shortness of breath at night, which would occasionally awaken him from sleep. At about the same time, he developed bilateral lower extremity swelling.

Over the course of the last year, he has been seen by his primary care physician and a nephrologist. An echocardiogram was obtained which showed normal left ventricular function and pharmacological myocardial perfusion imaging was unremarkable. He was treated with a diuretic which provided some improvement. Over the last several months, however, he has become progressively less responsive to the diuretic medication despite escalating doses.

He denies any recent illnesses, fevers, chills, sweats, arthritis, or additional symptoms. He specifically denies chest pain and states his only limitation to activity is shortness of breath.

Physical exam was notable for heart rate of 90 bpm, respirations of 12 per minute, blood pressure of 122/83 mmHg, and oxygen saturation of 98% on 2 l/min of oxygen by nasal cannula. The jugular veins were dilated to a height of 10 cm. Cardiovascular examination showed a regular rate and rhythm without murmur, gallop, or rub. His lungs were clear to auscultation bilaterally. Both upper

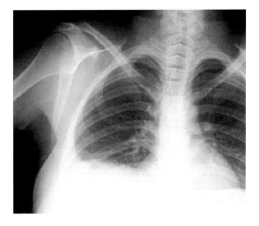

Figure 18.1 Chest x-ray.

extremities were warm and well perfused with no clubbing, cyanosis, or edema. The lower extremities had 2+ pretibial edema once compression stockings were removed.

Chest x-ray showed bilateral pleural effusions (R > L) but no airspace disease (Figure 18.1).

Right Heart Catheterization

Because of progressive symptoms despite medical management, the decision was made to proceed with right heart catheterization.

The major findings of the right heart catheterization were as follows:

- Right atrial pressures are markedly elevated (mean right atrial pressure is 17 mmHg) and contain prominent X and Y

Cardiology Board Review: ECG, Hemodynamic and Angiographic Unknowns, First Edition. Edited by George A. Stouffer.
© 2019 John Wiley & Sons Ltd. Published 2019 by John Wiley & Sons Ltd.

descents (labeled as having a "W" sign) (Figure 18.2). This filling pattern can be seen in various conditions including constrictive pericarditis, restrictive cardiomyopathy, and right ventricular infarction. The elevated right atrial pressures provide a hemodynamic explanation for the lower extremity edema.

- The prominent Y descent on right atrium (RA) tracing is characteristic of a condition in which early diastolic filling is important. The X descent is also preserved consistent with a cardiac condition in which ventricular filling after atrial contraction is also important. Lastly, note that the RA pressure does not decrease with inspiration (i.e. Kussmaul's sign). This finding suggests that intrathoracic pressure is not being communicated to intrapericardial space.
- The right ventricular waveform has a characteristic square root sign due to the rapid rise in early diastolic pressure prior to reaching the constraining effects of the rigid pericardium (Figure 18.3).
- Pulmonary artery pressures were unremarkable (Figure 18.4).

Simultaneous Right and Left Heart Catheterization

Because the diastolic pressures were elevated with features consistent with constrictive pericarditis or restrictive cardiomyopathy, left heart catheterization was performed and simultaneous left and right ventricular pressures were measured.

Right ventricular and left ventricular diastolic pressures are similar (Figure 18.5). The premature ventricular contraction (PVC) in the above tracing allows for a longer diastolic filling period and shows that the pressures do not separate even with prolonged diastole.

The next step was to evaluate for ventricular discordance. This is defined as inspiratory augmentation of right ventricle (RV) systolic pressure simultaneous with a decrease in left ventricle (LV) systolic pressure and occurs due to the effects of respiration on ventricular filling. Inspiration augments right heart filling at the expense of left heart filling. This is reflected as a drop in LV systolic pressure on particular cycles when the RV is rising (Figure 18.6).

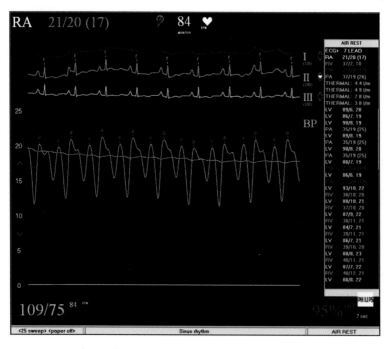

Figure 18.2 Right atrial pressure.

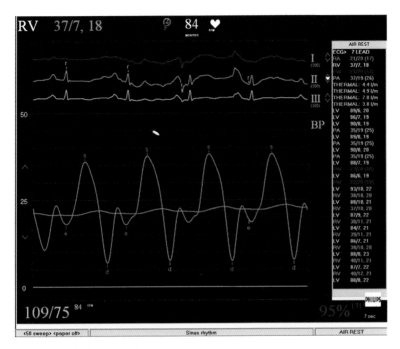

Figure 18.3 Right ventricular pressure.

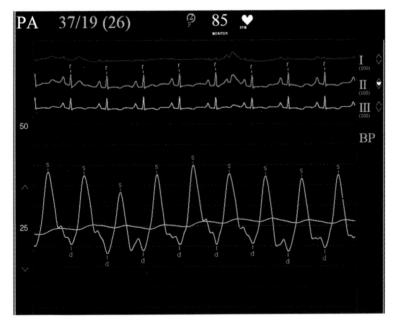

Figure 18.4 Pulmonary artery pressure.

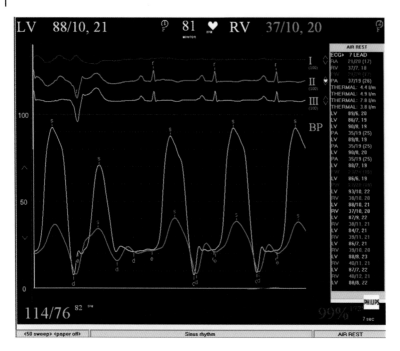

Figure 18.5 Simultaneous right ventricular and left ventricular pressures on a 100 mmHg scale with a fast sweep speed.

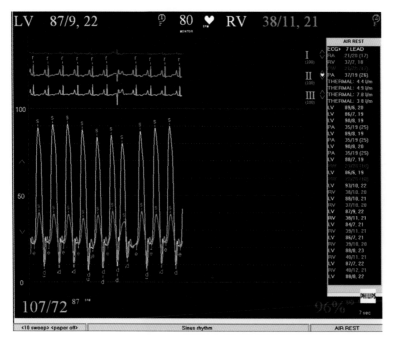

Figure 18.6 Simultaneous right ventricular and left ventricular pressures on a 100 mmHg scale with a slow sweep speed.

The right atrial and left ventricular diastolic pressures are also similar (Figure 18.7).

Cardiac output was 6.3 l/min by Assumed Fick method and 5.2 l/min by thermodilution. The coronary arteries were unremarkable.

In summary, the major findings at cardiac catheterization were:

1) Elevation of diastolic pressures.
2) Prominent X and Y descent on RA tracing.
3) Right and left ventricular diastolic pressures are elevated and similar.
4) LV diastolic pressures and RA pressures are similar.
5) Characteristic dip and plateau configuration to LV and RV pressure tracings.
6) RA pressure does not decrease with inspiration (i.e. Kussmaul's sign).
7) There was discordance of ventricular systolic pressures.

These findings are all consistent with constrictive pericarditis. Upon detailed questioning, he reported symptoms consistent with acute pericarditis five years ago. CT of the chest showed thickened pericardium with calcifications (Figure 18.8). He subsequently underwent pericardectomy with relief of symptoms and resolution of the lower extremity edema.

Constrictive Pericarditis

Clinically, constrictive pericarditis is generally a chronic disease with symptom progression over a period of years. The clinical presentation is that of right-sided heart failure and may resemble restrictive cardiomyopathy, cirrhosis, or *cor pulmonale* among other conditions. Occasionally patients will go for years without the correct diagnosis being made. Recently the widespread availability of newer cardiac diagnostic technologies and a change in the predominant etiologies of constriction has led to increasing recognition of subacute presentations that occur over a period of months rather than years.

A hallmark of constrictive pericarditis is the hemodynamic interdependence of the

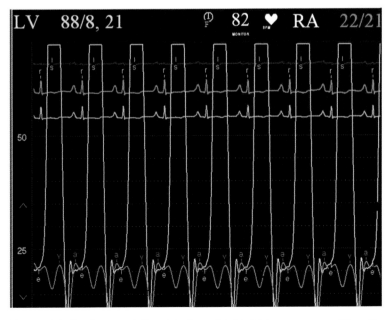

Figure 18.7 Simultaneous left ventricular and right atrial pressures on a 50 mmHg scale.

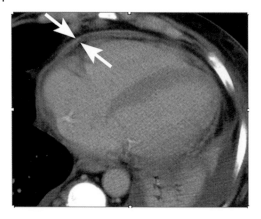

Figure 18.8 CT scan showing pericardial thickening.

cardiac chambers. In contrast to the normal heart where pressures in the cardiac chambers are independent (i.e. unrelated) during diastole, in constrictive pericarditis the stiff pericardium limits expansion of the cardiac chambers. The chambers can fill beyond a certain limited point only by compressing other chambers and thus the diastolic pressures equalize. Diastolic pressures in the RA, left atrium (LA), RV, and LV diastolic pressures are elevated and nearly identical.

The classic way of diagnosing constrictive pericarditis from hemodynamics is the finding that right and left ventricular diastolic pressures are elevated and similar. While comparison of left ventricular end diastolic pressure (LVEDP) and right ventricular end diastolic pressure (RVEDP) is the time honored way to evaluate for constrictive pericarditis, a comparison of mean pressures in the RA and the LA (or PCWP [pulmonary capillary wedge pressure]) may be more useful as such recordings are less subject to artifacts.

While the diagnosis of constrictive pericarditis in this patient became obvious after CT imaging of the pericardium, occasionally you will need to differentiate constrictive pericarditis from restrictive cardiomyopathy, two very different diseases sharing a similar hemodynamic profile. Both have as the primary hemodynamic abnormality altered mid to late diastolic filling of the ventricles leading to a syndrome of congestive heart failure. Often the heart failure is insidious in onset and predominantly right-sided. These syndromes may mimic many other disease entities and it is common for both conditions to go undiagnosed for years.

In the case of constrictive pericarditis, the impediment to filling is caused by the thickened unyielding pericardium. In restrictive cardiomyopathy the abnormality is a result of a poorly compliant myocardium that limits the ability of the ventricles to expand and accept the filling volume of the atria. Rarely there is overlap and both entities can coexist (e.g. radiation-induced myopericardial disease). The possibility of constriction or restriction should be entertained in any patient presenting with heart failure and normal systolic function (although systolic function will decline as restrictive cardiomyopathy progresses) particularly when other causes of this entity are not present.

Further Reading

Miranda, W.R. and Oh, J.K. (2017). Constrictive pericarditis: a practical clinical approach. *Progress in Cardiovascular Diseases* 59 (4): 369–379.

Stouffer, G.A. Constrictive Pericarditis in Cardiovascular Hemodynamics for the Clinician. 2nd Edition. Blackwell Publishing.

Welch, T.D. (2018). Constrictive pericarditis: diagnosis, management and clinical outcomes. *Heart* 104 (9): 725–731.

Case 19: A Clinical Application of Coronary Physiology

A 57-year-old male is referred to you for evaluation of exertional chest pain and dyspnea. Physical examination and ECG (electrocardiogram) are unremarkable. Echocardiography shows normal left ventricular systolic function. Because of worrisome symptoms, you decide to perform an exercise treadmill test which reproduces his symptoms and is notable for 2 mm of ST depression in multiple leads during stage 2 of the Bruce protocol. Coronary angiography shows a 90% stenosis at the ostium of the first obtuse marginal (OM) and a 70% stenosis in the mid-LAD (left anterior

descending) coronary artery (Figure 19.1). What is your next step?

Clinical Application of FFR

This is an excellent case to use fractional flow reserve (FFR) to determine which lesion(s) is responsible for the symptoms. FFR was performed to evaluate the OM lesion and the LAD lesion (Figures 19.2 and 19.3). Based upon the FFR results, the patient is most likely to achieve resolution of exertional symptoms with PCI (percutaneous coronary intervention) of the LAD.

(a)

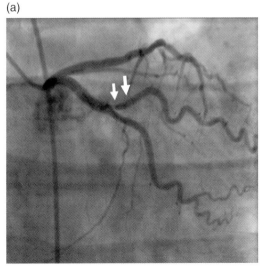

(b)

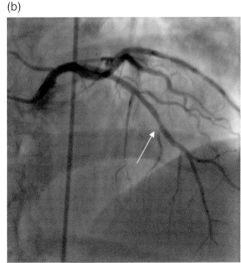

Figure 19.1 Left coronary angiography in an AP (anteroposterior) caudal view (a) and an AP cranial view (b). The thick arrows in panel (a) show the stenosis in the obtuse marginal and the thin arrow in panel (b) shows the stenosis in the LAD.

Cardiology Board Review: ECG, Hemodynamic and Angiographic Unknowns, First Edition. Edited by George A. Stouffer.
© 2019 John Wiley & Sons Ltd. Published 2019 by John Wiley & Sons Ltd.

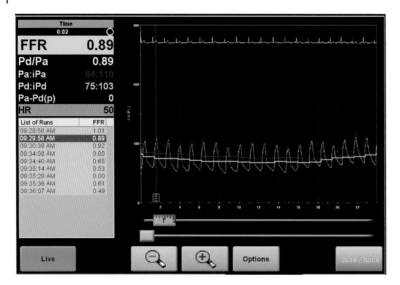

Figure 19.2 Fractional flow reserve (FFR) of OM.

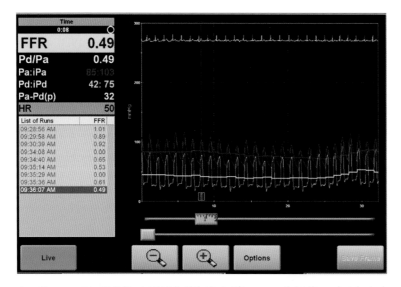

Figure 19.3 Fractional flow reserve (FFR) of LAD.

Basic Physiology of the Coronary Vasculature

Under basal conditions, the myocardium extracts 60–80% of the oxygen delivered to it via the coronary arteries. This is the highest oxygen consumption per tissue mass in the human body. In contrast to other tissues which respond to increased metabolic demand by increasing oxygen extraction or anaerobic metabolism, the myocardium relies on the ability to increase the oxygen supply via increasing coronary blood flow.

The coronary circulation can be broadly divided into the epicardial "conduit" arteries and the microvascular "resistance" vessels. In the healthy adult, the majority of myo-cardial flow regulation occurs by changes in microvascular resistance. Resistance is inversely proportional to flow and is affected by both extravascular and intravascular influences. The compressive force generated by the myocardium during systole is the pri-mary extravascular determinant of coronary flow. Systolic contraction causes a gradient of intramyocardial pressure, highest at the sub-endocardium and decreasing toward the subepicardium, resulting in compression of the microcirculation and flow impediment. Subsequently, the majority of microvascular coronary flow occurs during diastole. An increase in compressive forces, e.g. in situa-tions of increased contractility and wall stress, or reduced ventricular filling time associated with increased heart rate, can result in ischemia in the absence of epicardial obstruction.

Although extravascular compressive forces contribute significantly, the primary mecha-nism for dynamic, regionalized control of vascular resistance is in the microvasculature via regulating smooth muscle tone. Both mechanical forces and biochemical signals orchestrate vascular tone and their individual contributions differ by size of vessel. Mechanoreceptors respond to increased shear stress by causing vasodilation, mostly in the smaller arteries and larger arterioles measuring >100 μm in diameter. Intermediate-sized arterioles (50–100 μm) are capable of "myogenic control" whereby an increase or decrease in intraluminal pressure is counter-acted by the opposing change in vascular tone. Thus, when pressure in the vessel is high, smooth muscle cells contract to cause vasoconstriction; when pressure drops, smooth muscle cells relax to cause vasodi-lation. Lastly, a number of peptides, neuro-transmitters, and other small molecules act on the endothelium and underlying smooth muscle cells of all vessels, but particularly those less than 100 μm in diameter. These vasoactive compounds are products of cellular metabolism, sympathetic or para-sympathetic neural activity, or released by platelets. Prototypical examples include nitric oxide, adenosine, acetylcholine, and endothelin. It is important to note that the effect of vasoactive compounds critically relies on the health of the endothelium, which serves as an intermediary between signaling molecules in the bloodstream and the smooth muscle cells which wrap around blood vessels.

Autoregulation and Coronary Flow Reserve

The myocardium relies on a constant sup-ply of oxygenated blood. The ability of healthy coronary circulation to maintain constant flow over a range of perfusion pressures is called "autoregulation." The autoregulatory range has been experimen-tally measured to be 40–150 mmHg mean coronary pressure. Once coronary perfu-sion pressure drops below 40 mmHg, the coronary circulation becomes maximally dilated and coronary flow becomes directly proportional to pressure. The ability of the coronary circulation to increase flow when the vasculature is maximally dilated is referred to as the "coronary flow reserve" (CFR) (Gould et al. 1974). Normal CFR in humans when the vasculature is pharmaco-logically dilated is approximately 4–5 times the basal flow rate.

Autoregulation and CFR are clinically important in the context of increased meta-bolic demand on the heart, particularly in the presence of epicardial coronary artery disease (CAD). Under an increased workload and therefore oxygen demand, the coro-nary microcirculation vasodilates to allow increased myocardial blood flow. This flow reserve allows for the maintenance of myo-cardial perfusion without ischemia. However, atherosclerotic plaque in the epicardial coro-nary arteries results in a fixed resistance to flow and subsequently decreases pressure distal to the stenosis. Stenosis less than 90% of lumen diameter is unlikely to cause ischemia at rest because autoregulation and vasodilation allow for adequate flow maintenance. However, when oxygen demand increases above basal levels, the ability to increase coronary blood flow becomes very sensitive to stenosis severity. Lesions up to 50% of lumen diameter have minimal impact on CFR and adequate flow can be maintained even under increased workload or pharmacologically induced vasodilation. However, as stenosis severity increases above 50% lumen diameter, relaxation of vasodilatory reserve is required to maintain flow even at rest and therefore response to pharmacological vasodilation or exercise is blunted, leading to ischemia.

CFR can be directly measured in the catheterization lab with guidewires capable of measuring Doppler velocity. Assuming coronary diameter remains constant at a given point in the vessel, blood velocity is directly proportional to flow (flow = velocity × cross-sectional area). Flow during maximal hyperemia relative to basal flow at that point is calculated as the CFR. However, measurement of CFR by Doppler velocimetry is affected by conditions that raise basal blood flow (e.g. tachycardia, fever, anemia), and depends on the health of the microcirculation. Diabetes, hypertension, renal disease, and prior myocardial infarction can have detrimental effects on the coronary microcirculation globally or regionally. Additionally, measurement of CFR is technically difficult. Relative CFR is conceptually and technically similar, but overcomes the limitations of absolute CFR measurement by comparing the ratio of CFR in a diseased vessel to that of a healthy nonstenotic vessel. A major assumption for the application of relative CFR is that microcirculation function is uniform throughout the myocardium, which may not be the case in hearts which have sustained prior infarction. Relative CFR is the basis for nuclear myocardial perfusion stress imaging wherein relative differences in tracer uptake at stress versus rest are compared to normal regions of the heart.

Fractional Flow Reserve

Invasive measurements of intracoronary flow are technically challenging and "normal" versus "abnormal" flow measurements have been difficult to establish. The development of 0.014 in. guidewires with pressure transducers has allowed the adoption of pressure-derived estimation of CFR in a coronary artery. At maximum vasodilation, flow in a vessel is directly proportional to pressure. FFR represents the proportion of maximal flow in a given vessel that can be achieved in the presence of a stenosis within that vessel (Pijls et al. 1993). FFR is measured as the ratio of pressure distal to a stenosis ($P_{distal} - P_{wedge}$) to coronary driving pressure proximal to the stenosis ($P_{aorta} - P_{wedge}$) at maximum vasodilation induced by intravenous or intracoronary adenosine. P_{wedge} is the wedge pressure distal to a stenosis and accounts for pressure within the collateral circulation and coronary venous system. Although P_{wedge} is often assumed to be zero, variation in flow via the collateral circulation can affect FFR measurement (Iqbal et al. 2010; Toth et al. 2016).

FFR carries a Class 1a recommendation for guiding revascularization in angiographically intermediate coronary stenoses (50–70% stenosis) in patients with stable angina. The FFR value indicating a hemodynamically significant stenosis was defined by study of patients with stable angina, single-vessel CAD, and abnormal stress test who underwent balloon angioplasty (Pijls et al. 1995). FFR was measured before and after angioplasty and patients received a follow-up stress test within one week after intervention. Patients with subsequent normalization of stress test after intervention (i.e. successful angioplasty) had post-angioplasty FFR > 0.75 as compared to pre-angioplasty FFR < 0.75. This indicates that a FFR < 0.75, indicating reduction of coronary pressure of 25% or more due to a stenosis, can reliably discriminate lesions that are significant enough to cause ischemia.

The use of FFR to assess hemodynamic significance of vessel stenosis as a guide for intervention has been validated in several clinical trials. Three randomized trials have evaluated FFR in patients with stable CAD. DEFER showed that patients with single-vessel disease and stenosis with FFR > 0.75 can safely be treated with medical therapy alone, and in fact, have significantly lower event rates compared to those that received PCI and medical therapy after 15 years of follow up (Bech et al. 2001). In a second study, patients with multi-vessel disease and FFR-guided PCI had lower adverse event rates and similar symptomatic improvement after one year compared to angiography-guided PCI (FAME) (Tonino et al. 2009), and a follow up study showed that FFR-guided PCI reduced the need for urgent revascularization compared with medical therapy alone (FAME 2) (De Bruyne et al. 2012; De Bruyne et al. 2014) It should be noted that FAME and FAME 2 established the currently accepted "cutoff" for FFR of > 0.80.

The use of FFR-guided PCI of nonculprit arteries has been evaluated in randomized trials of patients with ST elevation myocardial infarction (STEMI). The DANAMI-3-PRIMULTI and Compare-Acute studies both showed that FFR-guided PCI of the nonculprit artery significantly reduced adverse events at one year, driven primarily by a decreased need for urgent revascularization. FFR can also be used to evaluate multiple discrete stenoses within the same vessel, although it is important to note that hemodynamic interactions exist between stenoses and that the simplified FFR equation above cannot always be used (Pijls et al. 2000).

Instantaneous wave-free ratio (iFR) utilizes the wave free period in diastole to make a pressure-only assessment of the hemodynamic significance of coronary stenoses without the need for pharmacological vasodilation (e.g. adenosine). Two large, prospective, randomized trials have demonstrated the noninferiority of iFR when compared with FFR for guiding revascularization (Davies et al. 2017; Götberg et al. 2017; Bhatt 2018).

References

Bech, G.J., De Bruyne, B., Pijls, N.H.J. et al. (2001). Fractional flow reserve to determine the appropriateness of angioplasty in moderate coronary stenosis: a randomized trial. *Circulation* 103 (24): 2928–2934.

Bhatt, D.L. (2018). Fractional flow reserve measurement for the physiological assessment of coronary artery stenosis severity. *JAMA* 320 (12): 1275–1276. https://doi.org/10.1001/jama.2018.10683.

Davies, J.E., Sen, S., Dehbi, H.M. et al. (2017). Use of the instantaneous wave-free ratio or fractional flow reserve in PCI. *The New England Journal of Medicine* 376: 1824–1834.

De Bruyne, B., Fearon, W.F., Pijls, N.H.J. et al. (2014). Fractional flow reserve-guided PCI for stable coronary artery disease. *The New England Journal of Medicine* 371 (13): 1208–1217. https://doi.org/10.1056/NEJMoa1408758. Epub 2014 Sep 1.

De Bruyne, B., Pijls, N.H.J., Kalesan, B. et al. (2012). Fractional flow reserve-guided PCI versus medical therapy in stable coronary disease. *The New England Journal of Medicine* 367 (11): 991–1001. https://doi.org/10.1056/NEJMoa1205361. Epub 2012 Aug 27.

Götberg, M., Christiansen, E., Gudmundsdottir, I.J. et al. (2017). Instantaneous wave-free ratio versus fractional flow reserve to guide PCI. *The New England Journal of Medicine* 376: 1813–1823.

Gould, K.L., Lipscomb, K., and Hamilton, G.W. (1974). Physiologic basis for assessing critical coronary stenosis. Instantaneous flow response and regional distribution during coronary hyperemia as measures of coronary flow reserve. *The American Journal of Cardiology* 33 (1): 87–94.

Iqbal, M.B., Shah, N., Khan, M. et al. (2010). Reduction in myocardial perfusion territory and its effect on the physiological severity of a coronary stenosis. *Circulation Cardiovascular Interventions* 3 (1): 89–90. https://doi.org/10.1161/CIRCINTERVENTIONS.109.904193.

Pijls, N.H., De Bruyne, B., Bech, G.J.W. et al. (2000). Coronary pressure measurement to assess the hemodynamic significance of serial stenoses within one coronary artery: validation in humans. *Circulation* 102 (19): 2371–2377.

Pijls, N.H., Van Gelder, B., Van der Voort, P. et al. (1995). Fractional flow reserve. A useful index to evaluate the influence of an epicardial coronary stenosis on myocardial blood flow [see comments]. *Circulation* 92 (11): 3183–3193.

Pijls, N.H., van Son, J.A., Kirkeeide, R.L. et al. (1993). Experimental basis of determining maximum coronary, myocardial, and collateral blood flow by pressure measurements for assessing functional stenosis severity before and after percutaneous transluminal coronary angioplasty. *Circulation* 87 (4): 1354–1367.

Tonino, P.A., De Bruyne, B., Pijls, N.H.J. et al. (2009). Fractional flow reserve versus angiography for guiding percutaneous coronary intervention. *The New England Journal of Medicine* 360 (3): 213–224. https://doi.org/10.1056/NEJMoa0807611.

Toth, G.G., De Bruyne, B., Rusinaru, D. et al. (2016). Impact of right atrial pressure on fractional flow reserve measurements: comparison of fractional flow reserve and myocardial fractional flow reserve in 1,600 coronary Stenoses. *JACC Cardiovascular Interventions* 9 (5): 453–459. https://doi.org/10.1016/j.jcin.2015.11.021. Epub 2016 Feb 17.

Case 20: An Asymptomatic Patient with a Very Unusual ECG

A vascular surgeon asks your opinion on an abnormal ECG (electrocardiogram) in a 39-year-old patient with end-stage renal disease. The patient has recently moved to the area and was referred to the surgeon for revision of dialysis access. The ECG was done as a routine preoperative assessment (Figure 20.1). The patient has no cardiac complaints.

Dextrocardia

The ECG is from a patient with dextrocardia. The two most prominent features in an ECG of a dextrocardia are the P wave axis and the morphology of the QRS waves of the precordial leads. In the normal heart with normal sinus rhythm, the P wave axis (determined from the limb leads) varies from 0 to +75° (i.e. directed inferiorly and leftward). The P wave is always upright in leads I and II. An ECG showing marked right-axis deviation of the P wave (negative in aVL and lead I) and low voltage in leads V_4 through V_6 should prompt consideration of dextrocardia. Atrial depolarization, and thus P wave axis, will be rightward in dextrocardia. In the precordial leads, there will be reverse R wave progression with the R wave being tallest in V1 and progressively decreasing in

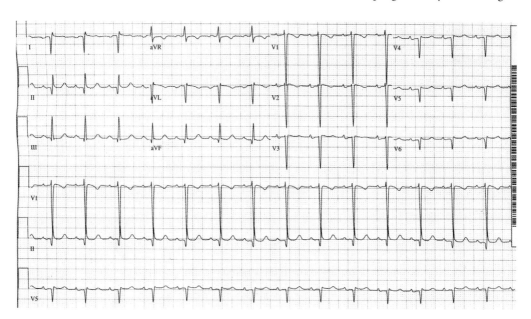

Figure 20.1 ECG on presentation.

Cardiology Board Review: ECG, Hemodynamic and Angiographic Unknowns, First Edition. Edited by George A. Stouffer.
© 2019 John Wiley & Sons Ltd. Published 2019 by John Wiley & Sons Ltd.

amplitude in leads V2 to V6. Other ECG findings which should prompt the thought of dextrocardia include: (i) a net positive QRS vector in AVR; (ii) an extreme rightward QRS axis (between –90 and –180°); and (iii) a tall R wave in V1.

Dextrocardia (from Latin dexter-, on the right-hand side, and Greek kardia-, heart) is a rare condition in which the heart is situated on the right side of the chest. There are various clinical scenarios that can lead to dextrocardia including: (i) the heart is shifted to the right side of the chest by factor extrinsic to the heart (e.g. the scimitar syndrome with hypoplasia of the right lung); (ii) rotational abnormalities of the cardiac loop during development (dextroversion; e.g. single ventricle or Cantrell syndrome); and (iii) dextrocardia associated with situs inversus in which the abdominal organs are also transposed. About one-third of the patients with situs inversus

will have heart malformations such as ventricular septal defect, atrial septal defect, Tetralogy of Fallot, tricuspid atresia, pulmonary stenosis, single ventricle, or complete or corrected transposition of the great arteries. Kartagener's syndrome consists of situs inversus, sinusitis, and bronchiectasis. Approximately two-thirds of people with dextrocardia and situs inversus are well, have structurally normal hearts, and live a normal lifespan.

Be aware of "pseudodextrocardia" in which the right arm and left arm leads are reversed. This will lead to "rightward" P wave and QRS axes. In general, P wave and QRS that are both predominantly negative in lead I generally only occur in two conditions: reversed arm leads or dextrocardia. A clue to the diagnosis of limb lead reversal in this setting is that the precordial wave voltage will generally appear normal.

Further Reading

Stout, K.K., Daniels, C.J., Aboulhosn, J.A. et al. (2018). 2018 AHA/ACC guideline for the Management of Adults with Congenital Heart Disease: a report of the American College of Cardiology/American Heart Association Task Force on Clinical Practice Guidelines. *Circulation* pii: S0735-1097(18)36846-3. https://doi.org/10.1016/j.jacc.2018.08.1029.

Case 21: Is This a STEMI?

A 42-year-old man presents to the Emergency Department with worsening chest pain. The patient has no history of heart disease and no risk factors for coronary artery disease except that his maternal grandfather had a myocardial infarction at 52 years of age. His chest pain is exacerbated by arm movement and reproducible on palpation.

Physical examination is remarkable for a blood pressure of 150/96 mmHg, pulse rate of 60 bpm, and oxygen saturation of 98% on room air. His lungs are clear and his cardiovascular examination is normal.

The ECG technician brings you the following ECG (Figure 21.1) and alerts you that the automated reading is for an anterior ST elevation myocardial infarction (STEMI). The nurse wants to know whether to activate the STEMI team. What is your diagnosis?

Early Repolarization

This ECG demonstrates the findings of early repolarization with J point elevation and ST segment elevation in leads I, II, AVF, and

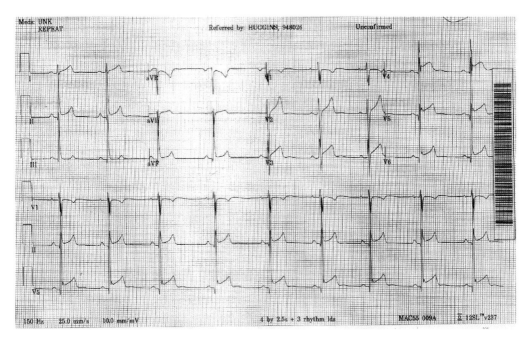

Figure 21.1 ECG on presentation.

Cardiology Board Review: ECG, Hemodynamic and Angiographic Unknowns, First Edition. Edited by George A. Stouffer. © 2019 John Wiley & Sons Ltd. Published 2019 by John Wiley & Sons Ltd.

V2–V6. Early repolarization is generally defined as J point elevation (elevation of the QRS–ST junction), slurring or notching of the J point, and ST segment elevation of at least 0.1 mV from baseline. The location of the maximal ST elevation in early repolarization is variable with the most common site being chest leads V_3 and V_4. Maximal ST elevation can, however, occur laterally (leads I, aVL, V_5, and V_6), inferiorly (leads II, III, and aVF), or anteriorly (leads V_1 and V_2).

Early repolarization is a common ECG variant being found in 1 to 7% of individuals. It is more common in young individuals, males, athletes, and African-Americans. Dynamic changes may occur in the width and height of the wave. For example, interventions that increase heart rate, such as exercise testing or isoproterenol infusion, generally reduce or eliminate early repolarization while agents that slow heart rate, such as beta blockers, will accent ST elevation in these patients.

Early repolarization has historically been considered benign although studies have linked early repolarization changes in the inferolateral leads to sudden cardiac death. A study by Haïssaguerre et al. found early repolarization in the inferolateral leads in 64 of 206 patients (31%) who were resuscitated after idiopathic ventricular fibrillation (Haïssaguerre et al. 2008).

Early repolarization can be confused with acute myocardial infarction or pericarditis. Several criteria can be used to identify patients with early repolarization although none are 100% accurate. These include: (i) absence of chest pain; (ii) young age; (iii) widespread ST elevation; (iv) marked J-point elevation; (v) concavity of initial upsloping portion of ST segment; (vi) notching or irregular contour of J point; (vii) prominent, concordant T waves; and (viii) current ECG is unchanged from prior ECGs. Distinguishing pericarditis from early repolarization may be difficult, although serial ECGs over several days may be helpful. In early repolarization the ST segments remain constant whereas, in general, the ECG in patients with acute pericarditis evolves over time.

Bibliography

Haïssaguerre, M., Derval, N., Sacher, F. et al. (2008). Sudden cardiac arrest associated with early repolarization. *New England Journal of Medicine* 358 (19): 2016–2023.

Macfarlane, P.W., Antzelevitch, C., Haïssaguerre, M. et al. (2015). The early repolarization pattern: a consensus paper. *Journal of the American College of Cardiology* 66 (4): 470–477.

Priori, S.G. and Napolitano, C. (2018). J-wave syndromes: electrocardiographic and clinical aspects. *Cardiac Electrophysiology Clinics* 10 (2): 355–369.

Case 22: Rapidly Progressive Dyspnea, Abdominal Fullness, and Nausea

A 55-year-old female with a history of osteo-arthritis presented with a five-day history of progressive dyspnea, abdominal fullness, and nausea. Cardiac exam showed normal S1 and S2 with no murmurs, rubs, or gallops. She had 1+ pitting edema and jugular venous distension to 10 cm with the head at 45°. Respiratory exam was remarkable for bibasilar crackles with no wheez-ing. Chest x-ray demonstrated pulmonary edema and an ECG was remarkable for nonspecific interventricular conduction delay. The MB frac-tion of creatine kinase (CK-MB) and troponin were elevated. Her thyroid-stimulating hormone (TSH) level was within normal limits and HIV (human immunodeficiency virus) testing was negative. Infectious serologies (coxsackie A and B, Lyme, HIV, EBV [Epstein-Barr virus], HSV [herpes simplex virus]) returned nega-tive but an antinuclear antibody was positive.

Echocardiography showed severe left ven-tricular systolic dysfunction with an ejection fraction of 15 to 20% and 3+ mitral regurgi-tation. Heart catheterization revealed normal coronary arteries but significantly elevated filling pressures.

Endomyocardial biopsy specimen is shown below (Figure 22.1). What is the most likely diagnosis?

Giant Cell Myocarditis

The clinical course is consistent with giant cell myocarditis (GCM) and the biopsy shows prominent myocyte necrosis with a diffuse inflammatory infiltrate.

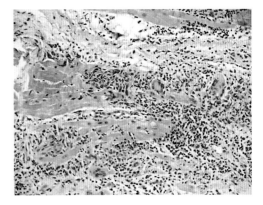

Figure 22.1 Myocardial biopsy stained with hematoxylin–eosin.

GCM is an inflammatory disease of the myocardium associated with myocyte necrosis and cardiac dysfunction of nonis-chemic origin. GCM is a rare and frequently fatal type of myocarditis that mainly affects young and otherwise healthy individuals. Failure to rapidly diagnose and treat GCM with a combination of immunosuppressive agents is associated with a median survival of 5.5 months from symptom onset.

Idiopathic GCM is a nonviral type of auto-immune myocarditis that has been attributed to T lymphocyte-mediated inflammation. Although the exact etiology of GCM is unknown, the association of GCM with various autoimmune disorders and tumors of immune cells, such as thymoma and lymphoma, suggests that dysregulated host immunity is responsible for GCM. The mixed inflammatory infiltrate of lympho-cytes, giant cells, and eosinophils results in a

Cardiology Board Review: ECG, Hemodynamic and Angiographic Unknowns, First Edition. Edited by George A. Stouffer.
© 2019 John Wiley & Sons Ltd. Published 2019 by John Wiley & Sons Ltd.

diffuse myocardial necrosis, which often results in fulminant deterioration of left ventricular systolic function.

Idiopathic GCM presents with signs and symptoms typical of heart failure and suspicion for myocarditis should increase in the absence of coronary disease. The clinical course is characterized by rapidly deteriorating left ventricular function refractory to standard heart failure therapies. GCM also has high rates of arrhythmias including ventricular arrhythmias and heart block. High-grade heart block is less common in other types of myocarditis and its presence may help to differentiate GCM from other causes of myocarditis.

EKG, cardiac enzymes, and echocardiography are initially helpful for narrowing the differential diagnoses but are not confirmatory for GCM. The gold standard for diagnosing all types of myocarditis is endomyocardial biopsy. However, performing an endomyocardial biopsy carries some risk and there is little standardization in sampling and interpreting biopsy results. In GCM, the biopsy will show an inflammatory myocardial infiltrate with necrosis and characteristic giant cells. In recent years, MRI has gained wider application as a noninvasive evaluation for myocarditis. A combination of T1 and T2 weighted images may reveal areas of myocarditis to strengthen a clinical suspicion or guide EMB for more accurate sampling.

GCM should be treated aggressively with combined immunosuppression. Patients treated with 2–4 immunosuppressive drugs, including cyclosporine, have approximately a 77% transplant-free survival. Patients should also receive standard heart failure and antiarrhythmic therapy. Anticoagulation should be used when there is evidence of systemic embolism or acute left ventricular thrombus. Patients with GCM should restrict the use of NSAIDS (nonsteroidal anti-inflammatory drugs), heavy alcohol consumption, and exercise to prevent the acceleration of viral replication.

Patients with GCM often need mechanical circulatory support when heart failure is intractable or cardiogenic shock does not respond to therapy. A biventricular device is used for mechanical circulatory support because of the incidence of progressive right ventricular failure and heart transplant listing. Although transplantation is an effective therapy for GCM, recurrence occurs in 25% of patients three years post-transplant.

Further Reading

Abdel-Aty, H., Boyé, P., Zagrosek, A. et al. (2005). Diagnostic performance of cardiovascular magnetic resonance in patients with suspected acute myocarditis: comparison of different approaches. *Journal of the American College of Cardiology* 45 (11): 1815–1822.

Cooper, L.T., Berry, G.J., and Shabetai, R. (1997). Idiopathic Giant-cell myocarditis – natural history and treatment. *The New England Journal of Medicine* 336 (26): 1860–1866.

Cooper, L.T., Hare, J.M., Tazelaar, H.D. et al. (2008). Usefulness of immunosuppression for Giant cell myocarditis. *The American Journal of Cardiology* 102 (11): 1535–1539.

Cooper, L.T., Keren, A., Sliwa, K. et al. (2014). The global burden of myocarditis: part 1: a systematic literature review for the global burden of diseases, injuries, and risk factors 2010 study. *Global Heart* 9 (1): 121–129.

Costanzo-Nordin, M.R., Reap, E.A., O'connell, J.B. et al. (1985). A nonsteroid anti-inflammatory drug exacerbates coxsackie B3 murine myocarditis. *Journal of the American College of Cardiology* 6 (5): 1078–1082.

Kandolin, R., Lehtonen, J., Salmenkivi, K. et al. (2013). Diagnosis, treatment, and outcome of giant-cell myocarditis in the era of combined immunosuppression. *Circulation Heart Failure* 6 (1): 15–22.

Khatib, R., Reyes, M.P., Smith, F. et al. (1990). Enhancement of coxsackievirus B4 virulence by indomethacin. *The Journal of Laboratory and Clinical Medicine* 116 (1): 116–120.

Maron, B.J., Udelson, J.E., Bonow, R.O. et al. (2015). Eligibility and disqualification recommendations for competitive athletes with cardiovascular abnormalities: task force 3: hypertrophic cardiomyopathy, Arrhythmogenic right ventricular cardiomyopathy and other cardiomyopathies, and myocarditis: a Scientif. *Journal of the American College of Cardiology* 66 (21): 2362–2371.

Moloney, E.D., Egan, J.J., Kelly, P. et al. (2005). Transplantation for myocarditis: a controversy revisited. *The Journal of Heart and Lung Transplantation* 24 (8): 1103–1110.

Rezkalla, S., Khatib, G., and Khatib, R. (1986). Coxsackievirus B3 murine myocarditis: deleterious effects of nonsteroidal anti-inflammatory agents. *The Journal of Laboratory and Clinical Medicine* 107 (4): 393–395.

Rosenstein, E.D., Zucker, M.J., and Kramer, N. (2000). Giant cell myocarditis: Most fatal of autoimmune diseases. *Seminars in Arthritis and Rheumatism* 30 (1): 1–16. https://doi.org/10.1053/SARH.2000.8367.

Wijetunga, M. and Rockson, S. (2002). Myocarditis in systemic lupus erythematosus. *The American Journal of Medicine* 113 (5): 419–423.

Case 23: A 40-Year-Old Man with Dyspnea on Exertion

A 40-year-old man with increasing dyspnea on exertion and lower extremity edema was referred to you for cardiac catheterization. Simultaneous measurement of pressures in the left ventricular (LV) apex and in the femoral artery were made with a PVC (premature ventricular contraction) (Figure 23.1a) and Valsalva maneuver (Figure 23.1b and c).

What is the diagnosis?

Hypertrophic Obstructive Cardiomyopathy

These hemodynamic tracings are consistent with hypertrophic obstructive cardiomyopathy (HOCM). Simultaneous measurement of LV apex and femoral artery pressures revealed no gradient under basal conditions. Initiation of a PVC elicited a Brockenbrough sign (Figure 23.1a) and having the patient perform a Valsalva maneuver precipitated a marked, transient increase in left ventricular outflow tract (LVOT) gradient (Figures 23.1b and c).

Hypertrophic cardiomyopathy (HCM) is the name given to a heterogeneous family of disorders characterized by genetic defects involving myocyte sarcomeric proteins. More than 1400 mutations in 11 genes encoding proteins have been described, with the most common defect being a mutation in the gene that encodes beta-myosin heavy chain. Defects in other genes encoding for sarcomeric proteins including troponin T, troponin I,

myosin light chains, alpha tropomyosin, and myosin-binding protein C have also been implicated in causing HCM. Inheritance is usually autosomal dominant with variable penetrance. Classically, HCM was defined by excessive septal hypertrophy (usually the width of the septum on echocardiography exceeding 1.5 cm) with or without the presence of outflow tract obstruction and even today most studies of HCM use echocardiographic, rather than genetic, criteria to determine eligibility. There are several anatomic variants of HCM that have been described. The most well-known phenotype from a hemodynamic standpoint is HOCM (also known as idiopathic hypertrophic subaortic stenosis). It was formally described as a distinct clinical entity in 1958 and consists of narrowing of the LVOT with ventricular contraction causing a dynamic pressure gradient. This anatomic pattern occurs in 25–50% of cases of HCM and will be the type of HCM that we concentrate on in this chapter.

Hemodynamics

Outflow tract obstruction in patients with HOCM is "dynamic," which means the resistance to flow changes depending on filling pressures, afterload (e.g. aortic pressure), and force of contractility. LVOT obstruction changes in severity depending on the force of systolic contraction and the dimensions of the LV (in contrast to aortic stenosis which is a fixed obstruction since it is valvular and not

Cardiology Board Review: ECG, Hemodynamic and Angiographic Unknowns, First Edition. Edited by George A. Stouffer.
© 2019 John Wiley & Sons Ltd. Published 2019 by John Wiley & Sons Ltd.

(a)

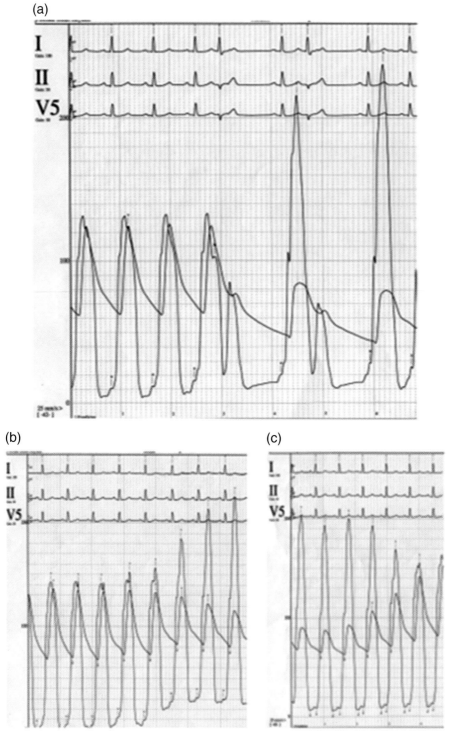

(b)   (c)

Figure 23.1 (a) Simultaneous left ventricular (LV) and femoral artery pressures; (b) and (c) Simultaneous LV and femoral artery pressures during Valsalva maneuver.

Table 23.1 Hemodynamic findings in HOCM.

Spike and dome configuration of arterial pulse	On aortic pressure tracing, there is a rapid rise during systole which is followed by a mild drop in pressure and then a secondary peak
Systolic intraventricular pressure gradient	Simultaneous intraventricular and aortic pressure tracings will show a difference in maximum systolic pressure at rest and/or with provocation
Diastolic dysfunction	LV end-diastolic pressure will be elevated, the rapid phase of LV filling will be prolonged and atrial contribution to LV filling will be accentuated
Brockenbrough sign	Aortic pulse pressure fails to widen during a post-extrasystolic beat

Source: used with permission from Cardiovascular Hemodynamics for the Clinician; 2nd ed., George Stouffer.

muscular). Thus, patients with HOCM may not have any obstruction while at rest but may develop significant pressure gradients during any activity which increases the force of cardiac contraction (e.g. exercise, emotional stress) or at times when their LV is smaller because of incomplete filling (e.g. dehydration). This obstruction can cause pressure gradients of greater than 100 mmHg and is thought to be one etiology of exercise-induced syncope in these patients (another potential etiology is arrhythmias).

LVOT gradients can be provoked using methods that decrease filling pressures and stroke volume (e.g. Valsalva maneuver or nitroglycerin) or methods that increase the force of contraction (post-PVC or iso-proterenol infusion). Dobutamine should be avoided as it can cause subaortic pressure gradients in normal hearts due to catecholamine stimulant effects.

A variable finding in HOCM is that the dynamic nature of the outflow tract obstruction causes a "spike and dome" configuration of the aortic or peripheral pulse (Table 23.1). This is known as a bisferiens pulse, a name derived from Latin: *Bis* (two) and *Feriere* (to beat). The bisferiens pulse is characterized by an initial rapid rise in aortic pressure (spike), followed by a slight drop in pressure (dip), and then a secondary peak (dome), and is most prominent in central aortic pressure but can also be transmitted to the carotids. It is enhanced by maneuvers that increase intraventricular pressure gradients (e.g. following a PVC or by the Valsalva maneuver) and in patients with obstruction only during provocation, a normal-appearing pressure tracing will often be replaced by the spike and dome during provocative maneuvers. Bisferiens pulse should be not confused with the dicrotic pulse, a pulse with an exaggerated dicrotic wave. A bisferiens pulse is most commonly associated with HOCM but can also be seen in severe aortic regurgitation.

The Brockenbrough–Braunwald–Morrow sign was originally described in 1961. This sign is present if the aortic pulse pressure falls in the first normal beat post-PVC in HOCM. While originally thought to be specific for HOCM, it has since been described in some cases of aortic stenosis.

Further Reading

Maron, B.J. (2018). Clinical course and management of hypertrophic cardiomyopathy. *New England Journal of Medicine* 379 (7): 655–668.

Maron, B.J., Ommen, S.R., Semsarian, C. et al. (2014). Hypertrophic cardiomyopathy: present and future, with translation into contemporary cardiovascular medicine. *Journal of the American College of Cardiology* 64 (1): 83–99.

Case 24: A Recent Immigrant from Mexico with Complaints of Dyspnea

A 32-year-old female who lived in Mexico until several months ago presents to your Emergency Department with profound dyspnea. According to the patient, she has been treated for heart failure for the past five years. She has been told that she has heart problems since she was a child but has not been told a specific diagnosis. She was admitted to another hospital several weeks ago for "pneumonia" and was treated with Bilevel Positive Airway Pressure (BiPAP) and antibiotics.

On examination, she is a thin Hispanic female with blood pressure of 120/70mmHg, pulse rate of 80bpm, and oxygen saturation of 97% on room air. Jugular venous pulsation (JVP) is elevated at ~12cm. Her lungs are clear. The first heart sound is normal but the second heart sound is obscured by a continuous crescendo–decrescendo murmur heard best at the left upper sternal border. There is 2+ pitting edema in the lower extremities.

What clues does the ECG (Figure 24.1) provide in establishing a differential diagnosis?

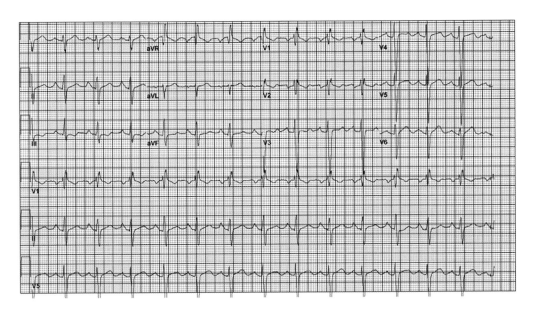

Figure 24.1 ECG on presentation.

Cardiology Board Review: ECG, Hemodynamic and Angiographic Unknowns, First Edition. Edited by George A. Stouffer.
© 2019 John Wiley & Sons Ltd. Published 2019 by John Wiley & Sons Ltd.

Patent Ductus Arteriosus

The ECG shows right axis deviation (RAD), right bundle branch block (RBBB), and right atrial enlargement. RAD in the frontal plane, large R waves in the right precordial leads, deep S waves in the left precordial leads, and a mild increase in QRS duration are consistent with right ventricular hypertrophy (RVH). These findings are suggestive of a lesion causing right ventricular volume or pressure overload.

In this individual, the cause was a patent ductus arteriosus (PDA). Other types of heart disease that would be in the differential diagnosis based on this ECG include congenital heart defects that result in left-to-right shunting, such as atrial septal defect or ventricular septal defect and acquired or congenital disorders that result in right ventricular pressure overload such as mitral stenosis, cor pulmonale, primary pulmonary hypertension, pulmonic stenosis, tetralogy of Fallot, and other rare types of congenital heart disease.

The ECG reflects the hemodynamic effects of the PDA. With a small PDA, a normal ECG is common. This ECG shows left atrial enlargement which is not uncommon in patients with a PDA with a moderate or large left-to-right shunt. Left ventricular hypertrophy (LVH) (with or without RVH) can also be seen in these cases. RVH on ECG generally indicates a large left-to-right-shunt with the development of pulmonary hypertension.

The ductus arteriosus connects the descending aorta (it usually originates just distal to the left subclavian artery) to the left pulmonary artery. In the fetus, blood flow via the ductus arteriosus is from the pulmonary artery to the aorta thus enabling blood to bypass the unexpanded lungs and enter the descending aorta for oxygenation in the placenta. At birth there is a decline of prostaglandin with the increase in PaO2 and the ductus arteriosus usually closes within a few days. If closure does not occur, blood can flow from the aorta to the pulmonary artery leading to increased pressure and volume in the pulmonary circulation. Symptoms depend on the size of the shunt, with large shunts having the possibly of leading to Eisenmenger's syndrome.

In this patient, cardiac catheterization demonstrated a PDA with a calculated shunt fraction (Qp/Qs) of 2.5. Cardiac output (Qs) as measured using the assumed Fick method was 9.1 l/min and pulmonary vascular resistance was 6.3 Wood units. An attempt was made to close the PDA percutaneously however it was too large for any existing closure device and the patient subsequently underwent successful surgical closure.

ECG Clues to the Presence of Hemodynamically Significant Congenital or Valvular Heart Disease in Young Adults

The 12 lead ECG can provide important clues to the presence of undiagnosed, hemodynamically significant cardiovascular disease in young adults (Table 24.1). The ECG has several limitations – it is neither sensitive nor specific and is rarely diagnostic of a specific condition. It is however readily available and when properly interpreted can prompt further evaluation (e.g. echocardiography) that will provide specific information as to the presence of congenital heart disease or valvular heart disease.

ECG patterns suggestive of hemodynamically important congenital or valvular heart disease reflect abnormalities of one of the cardiac chambers. Most commonly, these cardiovascular conditions will alter right heart pressures and/or volumes and thus lead to ECG changes reflective of right atrial abnormalities (RAA) or RVH. Less commonly, abnormal hemodynamics will affect the left atrium and/or left ventricle (LV) leading to ECG changes pointing to these chambers. In this chapter several ECG findings that may be clues to the presence of underlying cardiovascular disease in young adults will be discussed. These include:

- Tall R wave in lead V1
- RBBB
- RAD
- RVH

Table 24.1 Common ECG findings in adult patients with congenital heart disease. Note that the ECG findings are dependent upon the hemodynamic effects of the congenital heart defect.

	QRS Axis	QRS	RAA	RVH	LAA	LVH	Misc
Secundum ASD	Normal or RAD	RSR' in V1, IRBBB or RBBB	+				1AVB is common
Primum ASD	LAD	RSR' in V1			+		1AVB is common
Sinus venosus ASD							Ectopic atrial rhythm is common
PDA	Normal	Deep S wave in V1 +/– tall R waves in V5 and V6			+		
MS				+	+		
PS or PHTN	RAD		+	+			
VSD	RAD	RBBB	+	+	+	+	
Dextrocardia	RAD	Small R waves in left precordial leads		May have appearance of RVH			
Unrepaired TOF	RAD		+	+			

PDA = patent ductus arteriosus; ASD = atrial septal defect; VSD = ventricular septal defect; MS = mitral stenosis; PS = pulmonic stenosis; PHTN = pulmonary hypertension; TOF = tetralogy of Fallot; 1AVB = first-degree AV block.

- RAA
- LVH
- Left atrial abnormality

When interpreting an ECG in a young adult, two important caveats should be kept in mind. One is that "normal" ECG patterns change as we age. Many of the findings above are common in children but rare in adults. Since ECG changes with aging vary in different individuals, there will be some individuals where abnormal ECG findings reflect cardiovascular disease whereas the same pattern may reflect a nonpathologic, persistent juvenile ECG pattern in others.

Second, ECG patterns suggestive of cardiovascular disease may be present in well-conditioned athletes but do not necessarily reflect underlying pathology. ECG findings of LVH are common in athletes and can be a normal response to exercise and reversible with deconditioning. Also common are incomplete RBBB (14–31% of athletes), early repolarization, and bradycardia. These changes are more common in endurance sports (e.g. rowing or long-distance running) or sports with high peak level of activity (e.g. basketball or football). Note that the diagnosis of "athlete's heart" is one of exclusion and all athletes, most especially those with symptoms, should have a complete work-up before attributing an abnormal ECG to cardiac conditioning.

Findings Suggestive of Abnormal Right Heart Hemodynamic

Pronounced R Wave in Lead V1

V1 is the lead closest to the RV and thus is one of the most sensitive indicators of right ventricular pressure or volume overload. A pronounced R wave in V1, in the presence of a normal QRS duration, is a common finding in children, especially those less than eight years. The prevalence is less in older children, lesser still in young adults, and rare in older adults. An R wave in V1 is generally considered abnormal when >6 mm (Figure 24.1). Also abnormal are small S waves (<2 mm) and/or large R prime (R') waves (>10 mm). Another

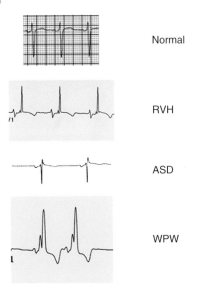

Normal

RVH

ASD

WPW

Figure 24.2 Lead V1 in various conditions (ASD = atrial septal defect; RVH = right ventricular hypertrophy; WPW = Wolff–Parkinson–White).

useful indicator is the R/S ratio which is >1 in less than 1% of adults. Any of these findings should prompt consideration of RVH, especially in the presence of RAD. A pronounced R wave in V1 can be a normal variant, especially in younger adults. Other causes of a large R wave in V1 include lead misplacement, posterior myocardial infarction (MI), Duchenne's Muscular Dystrophy, Type A pre-excitation pattern (Wolff-Parkinson-White), and displacement of the heart due to pulmonary disease (Figure 24.2).

Right Bundle Branch Block

RBBB can be a marker of dilation of the RV and thus may reflect cardiovascular disease leading to RV volume or pressure overload. The prevalence of RBBB increases with age and it is unusual in young adults. In a study of 237 000 airmen under the age of 30 years, the incidence of RBBB was only 0.2%. In the presence of RBBB, the predominant ST-T vector is usually discordant in the right precordial leads and upright in the left precordial leads and in leads I and aVL. Variations in this pattern may be another signal of underlying cardiovascular disease.

The right bundle branch originates from the bundle of His, courses through the ventricular septum to the apex, and then proceeds to the RV free wall. RBBB reflects a delay in RV depolarization (via the right bundle branch), usually resulting in a large terminal R′ wave in V1 (RSR′) and a broad terminal S wave in leads T, aVL, and V6. The World Health Organization (WHO)/International Society and Federation for Cardiology Task Force criteria for the diagnosis of RBBB include: QRS duration >120 ms; an RSR′ pattern in leads V1 and V2; S wave longer than 40 ms in V6 and I; normal R peak time in leads V5 and V6 but ≥50 ms in V1. The term incomplete right bundle branch block is used to describe the ECG when changes such as those described are present but the QRS interval is between 80 and 110 ms. Note that the QRS axis is unaffected by RBBB and thus axis deviation (either right or left) should prompt consideration of conditions that result in axis deviation.

Right Axis Deviation

RAD is normal in infants and children but unusual in adults. In one study, an axis >105° was found in only 2% of "normals" between the ages of 20 and 30 years. RAD can reflect right heart pathology as a hypertrophied RV can generate forces that balance and/or exceed the electrical forces generated by the usually much larger LV. The combination of a large R wave in V1 and RAD is highly suggestive of RVH. Other conditions associated with RAD include arm lead reversal, left posterior hemiblock, lateral wall MI, or lung disease. RAD can also be a normal variant, especially in individuals who are tall and slender.

Right Ventricular Hypertrophy

In the normal heart, RV voltage is almost completely masked by LV voltage and thus prominent RV forces are unusual and suggestive of RVH. As the RV develops increased muscle mass (i.e. hypertrophies), electrical voltage generated by the RV increases. This produces progressive anterior and rightward displacement of the QRS vector. Increases in RV muscle mass can cause prolongation of RV depolarization resulting in an increase in the duration of the QRS complex. These changes become more pronounced as the degree of hypertrophy increases.

There are different types of ECG patterns which have, with various success, been correlated to different causes of RVH. The first type is associated with lesions causing pressure overload of the RV and is characterized by a tall R wave in V1. This pattern has been associated with congenital pulmonic stenosis, tetralogy of Fallot, primary pulmonary hypertension, and other conditions associated with RV outflow obstruction. A second type, characterized by an RSR′ pattern, is seen in conditions with RV volume overload such as atrial septal defect. Lastly, ECG evidence of RVH in the presence of lung disease is affected by the spatial orientation of the heart and is characterized by low R wave amplitude and a posteriorly and superiorly oriented QRS vector (Figure 24.3).

The sensitivity and specificity of the ECG diagnosis of RVH is limited and this has led to a proliferation of criteria for the diagnosis of RVH. The sensitivity and specificity of the different criteria vary depending on the particular study and the patient population but in general for all of these formulas, specificity is greater than sensitivity. There are numerous criteria for the diagnosis of RVH but it is probably necessary only to keep the most common criteria in mind.

Tall R-waves in RV leads; deep S-waves in LV leads

- R/S ratio in V1 > 1
- R wave in V1 > 7 mm
- S wave in V1 of less than 2 mm
- RSR′ in V1 with R′ > 10 mm
- S1S2S3 pattern
- R/S ratio in V5 or V6 < 1
- R wave in aVR of more than 5 mm

The ECG diagnosis of RVH is enhanced if there are other findings of right heart pathology in the presence of increased RV voltage. These include RAA, RAD, an increase in QRS duration, and/or ST and T wave abnormalities in

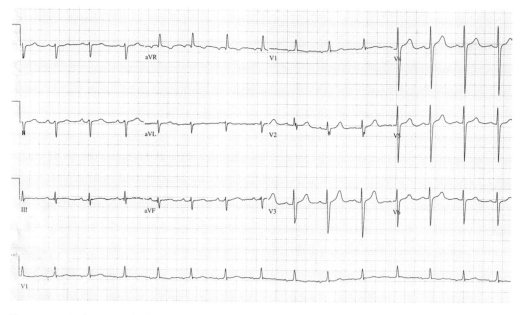

Figure 24.3 Right ventricular hypertrophy (RVH) in a patient with lung disease. Note the right axis deviation, relatively large R wave in V1, low limb lead voltage, relatively large R wave in aVR and deep S waves in the lateral precordial leads. This ECG is from an 18 year old man with cystic fibrosis.

the right precordial leads directed opposite to the predominant QRS direction (i.e. wide QRS/T angle). These findings are analogous to those which increase the likelihood of LVH in the presence of increased LV voltage.

Right Atrial Abnormality

Normally the P wave is formed by overlapping depolarization of the right and left atria leading to a smooth rounded wave less than 0.12 seconds in duration and less than 1 mm in height. The forces generated by right atrial depolarisation are directed anteriorly and inferiorly and produce the early part of the P wave. In the presence of right atrial enlargement, P wave amplitude increases although the overall duration of the P wave is usually not prolonged. As P-pulmonale progresses, the voltage in the P wave increases both from delayed activation of the right atrium causing simultaneous activation of the right and left atria and in the increase in right atrial tissue that is depolarizing.

P pulmonale is defined as tall (≥ 2.5 mV), peaked P waves in any of the inferior leads (II, III and aVF) with normal P wave duration (Figure 24.4). Less consistently, it can also include a positive deflection in the P wave in V1 or V2 of ≥ 1.5 mm. Remember that since the right atria depolarizes first, the first part of the P wave is indicative of the right atrium in V1. P-pulmonale is a marker of right atrial dilation or hypertrophy and can be seen in chronic obstructive pulmonary disease

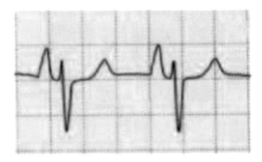

Figure 24.4 Right atrial abnormality.

(COPD), pneumonia, congenital heart disease, congestive heart failure, pulmonary emboli, asthma, or tricuspid valve disease.

The presence of an ectopic atrial rhythm can be a clue to congenital heart disease (e.g. sinus venosus atrial septal defect). The SA node is the normal pacemaker of the heart and is located in the posterior part of the right atrium at the junction of the superior vena cava. When the pacemaker function is controlled by the sinus node, P waves are positive in leads I, II, and aVF and negative in aVR (the normal P wave axis is 15–75°). An ectopic atrial rhythm means that the pacemaker function is now controlled by a focus within the atria (usually due to increased triggered automaticity). Normally the PR interval will remain within normal limits and the atrial rate will be below 100 beats per minute but the P wave morphology and axis will change. When the focus is lower in the atrium, the P wave in the inferior leads are inverted and the rhythm can be mistaken for an AV junctional rhythm.

Further Reading

Deen, J.F. and Jones, T.K. (2015 Nov). Shunt Lesions. *Cardiology Clinics.* 33 (4): 513–520, vii. https://doi.org/10.1016/j.ccl.2015.07.009. Epub 2015 Aug 22.

Stout, K.K., Daniels, C.J., Aboulhosn, J.A. et al. (2018). 2018 AHA/ACC Guideline for the Management of Adults With Congenital Heart Disease: A Report of the American College of Cardiology/American Heart Association Task Force on Clinical Practice Guidelines. *Journal of the American College of Cardiology* pii: S0735-1097(18)36845-1. https://doi.org/10.1016/j.jacc.2018.08.1028.

Case 25: New Onset Hypertension with Dyspnea and ECG Changes

You are asked to see a 39-year-old female with no significant past medical history who presented to the Emergency Department (ED) with worsening shortness of breath. She has no significant past medical history but reports several weeks of malaise, fatigue, and dyspnea. She came to the ED after awakening with a feeling of smothering.

On exam, she is dyspneic and diaphoretic. Blood pressure is 200/120 mmHg. She has bilateral rales and 2+ ankle edema. Her ECG is shown below. What are the important findings on the ECG (Figure 25.1)?

Hyperkalemia (with New Onset Renal Failure)

The magnitude of the electrolyte gradients across cell membranes has an important influence of depolarization and repolarization of myocardial cells. Thus it is no surprise that electrolyte abnormalities can have an effect, occasionally profound, on the ECG. Recognition of these changes can provide clues to diagnosing and treating potentially life-threatening conditions.

The most common ECG change with hyperkalemia is tall T waves, best seen in

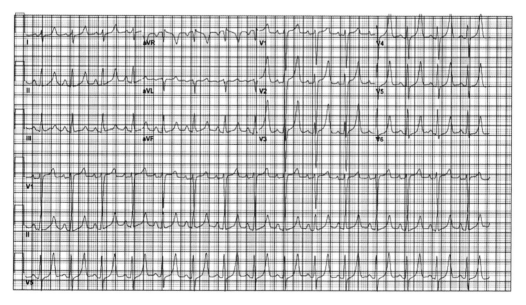

Figure 25.1 ECG on presentation.

Cardiology Board Review: ECG, Hemodynamic and Angiographic Unknowns, First Edition. Edited by George A. Stouffer.
© 2019 John Wiley & Sons Ltd. Published 2019 by John Wiley & Sons Ltd.

leads II, III, and V2–V4 (Table 25.1). Tall T waves are usually seen when the potassium concentration rises above 5.5–6.5 mmol/l, however only about one in five hyperkalemic patients will have the classic tall, symmetrically narrow and peaked T waves ("pinched" T waves); the rest will merely have large amplitude T waves. Hyperkalemia should be suspected when the amplitude of the T wave is greater than or equal to that of the R wave in more than one lead.

At higher potassium concentrations, the P wave widens and flattens and the PR segment lengthens (Table 25.2). As the concentration rises further, the P waves may disappear.

The QRS complex will begin to widen with a potassium concentration of 7.0–8.0 mmol/l. Unlike right or left bundle branch blocks, the QRS widening in hyperkalemia affects all portions of the QRS complex and not just the terminal forces. Severe untreated hyperkalemia can cause the QRS complex to merge with the T wave (a sine wave pattern), idioventricular rhythms, and asystolic cardiac arrest.

ST-segment elevation in leads V_1 and V_2 has been reported in severe hyperkalemia. Since dialysis corrects hyperkalemia and results in normalization of the ST segment elevation, this has been referred to in older literature as the "dialyzable current of injury."

The potassium level on initial presentation in this patient was 6.8 mmol/l. Six hours later following dialysis, the potassium level was 4.7 mmol/l (Figure 25.2). The patient was subsequently diagnosed with lupus nephritis.

Table 25.1 ECG changes associated with electrolyte abnormalities.

	Increased	Decreased
K^+	Tall, narrow, peaked T waves QRS prolongation Decreased amplitude of P waves Absent P waves ST segment elevation in V1 and V2 Sine wave appearance	ST segment depression Decreased T wave amplitude or T wave inversion Prominent U waves (mid precordial leads) QRS widening (children) Arrhythmias and AV block
Ca^+	Decrease in QTc (a short QT interval with minimal ST segment is characteristic of hypercalcemia) No change in morphology of P or T waves PR interval and QRS duration may be prolonged Arrhythmias are uncommon although AV block has been reported Can worsen digitalis toxicity Many patients with hypercalcemia develop hypokalemia	Prolongation of QTc P and T waves usually not affected QRS and PR duration usually not affected
Na^{++}	No effect	No effect
Mg^{++}	Minimal effects; extremely high serum magnesium levels may produce bradycardia or cardiac arrhythmias	Usually minimal effects on the ECG but can co-exist with hypokalemia. Torsades de pointes (multifocal ventricular tachycardia) may be precipitated.

Table 25.2 ECG changes in hyperkalemia.

Approximate serum potassium concentration (mEq/l)	ECG changes
5.5–6.5	Tall peaked T waves
6.5–7.5	Loss of P waves
7–8	Widening of QRS complexes
8–10	Sine wave, ventricular arrhythmias, asystole

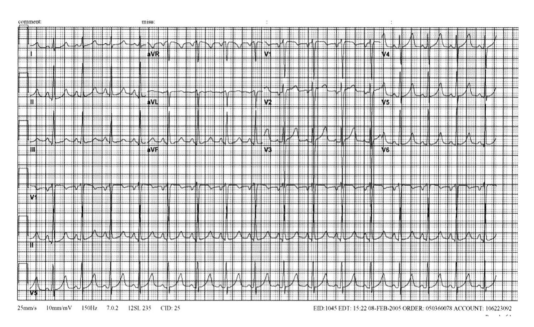

Figure 25.2 ECG in the patient after dialysis (K+ = 4.7 mmol/l).

Further Reading

El-Sherif, N. and Turitto, G. (2011). Electrolyte disorders and arrhythmogenesis. *Cardiology Journal* 18 (3): 233–245.

Mattu, A., Brady, W.J., and Robinson, D.A. (2000). Electrocardiographic manifestations of hyperkalemia. *The American Journal of Emergency Medicine* 18 (6): 721–729.

Case 26: A 52-Year-Old Woman on Hemodialysis Who Presents with Shortness of Breath and New ECG Changes

A 52-year-old female with a systemic lupus erythematosus who is on three times per week hemodialysis for end-stage renal disease presents to the local Emergency Department with complaints of shortness of breath, abdominal distention, and worsening lower extremity edema. She lives in another state and was visiting family in the area. She missed her most recent dialysis session. The Emergency Department physician was worried about the ECG and asks for your opinion.

On examination, she is an ill-appearing female with blood pressure of 174/102 mmHg, heart rate of 100 bpm, and oxygen saturation of 94% on room air. She has rales in the bases on her lung exam but her cardiovascular examination is unremarkable.

What does her ECG show (Figure 26.1)?

Hypocalcemia

The ECG shows findings consistent with hypocalcemia (her serum level of Ca was 7.8 mg/dl; normal range is 8.5–10.2 mg/dl). She had bone mineral disease and was receiving calcitriol with each dialysis but had missed her most recent dose.

Alterations in calcium levels predominantly alters phase 2 of the action potential

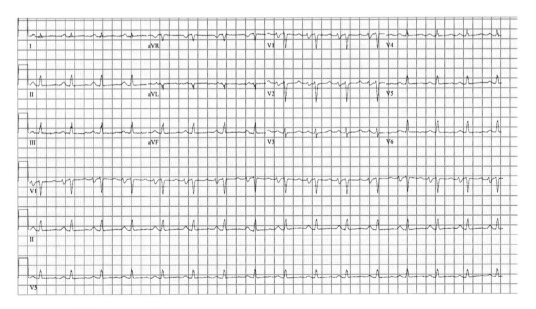

Figure 26.1 ECG on presentation.

Cardiology Board Review: ECG, Hemodynamic and Angiographic Unknowns, First Edition. Edited by George A. Stouffer.
© 2019 John Wiley & Sons Ltd. Published 2019 by John Wiley & Sons Ltd.

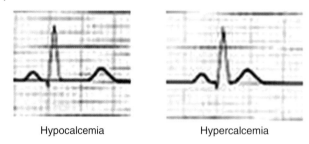

Hypocalcemia   Hypercalcemia

Figure 26.2 ECG changes in hypocalcemia and hypercalcemia.

resulting in shortening (hypercalcemia) or prolongation (hypocalcemia) of the QT interval (Figure 26.2). The influence on the QT interval is primarily due to a modification of the duration of the ST segment although both conditions can affect T wave morphology. Changes in calcium levels generally do not cause T wave changes because they do not affect phase 3 of the action potential, although there are case reports of altered T waves in hypocalcemia.

Hypercalcemia is associated with shortening of the QT interval (again, primarily due to shortening of the ST segment). At high calcium concentrations the duration of the T wave increases and the QT interval may then become normal. Prolongation of the PR and QRS intervals may also occur at high calcium concentrations. More rarely, second-degree or third-degree AV (atrioventricular) block and the appearance of Osborn waves (generally seen in hypothermia) have been reported.

QT prolongation can be seen in hypocalcemia and is primarily due to ST segment prolongation. The combination of hypocalcemia and hyperkalemia, which is seen most frequently in patients with renal insufficiency, produces a characteristic ECG pattern of tall, narrow T waves (from hyperkalemia) and ST segment prolongation (from hypocalcemia).

Further Reading

Diercks, D.B., Shumaik, G.M., Harrigan, R.A. et al. (2004). Electrocardiographic manifestations: electrolyte abnormalities. *The Journal of Emergency Medicine* 27 (2): 153–160.

El-Sherif, N. and Turitto, G. (2011). Electrolyte disorders and arrhythmogenesis. *Cardiology Journal* 18 (3): 233–245.

RuDusky, B.M. (2001). ECG abnormalities associated with hypocalcemia. *Chest* 119 (2): 668–668.

Case 27: A 42-Year-Old Man with Hypotension, Diarrhea, Vomiting, and ECG Changes

You are asked to evaluate the ECG on a 42-year-old male with hypertension who came to the Emergency Department because of weakness and fatigue. He was healthy until five days ago when he developed diarrhea and vomiting. The symptoms worsened three days ago and he has not eaten since that time but has continued to take his medications for hypertension which include hydrochlorothiazide and metoprolol. He gets dizzy when he stands and has been essentially bedbound for the last 24 hours.

On physical exam, he is ill appearing with a systolic blood pressure of 86/58 mmHg. What are the important findings from the ECG (Figure 27.1)?

Hypokalemia

ECG changes are rare with mild hypokalemia but may be present with more severe hypokalemia, especially if the individual has hypomagnesemia, coronary artery disease, or is taking a digitalis derivative (Table 27.1). These changes are primarily due to delayed ventricular repolarization and include decreased T wave amplitude, ST segment depression, prolongation of the QT interval, and accentuation of the U wave (Figure 27.1). A prominent U wave, in association with a small T wave in the setting of a prolonged QT interval, are findings that should raise the suspicion of hypokalemia.

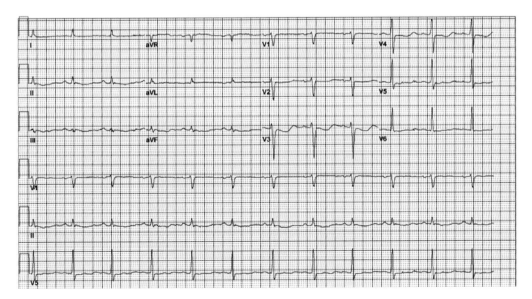

Figure 27.1 ECG on presentation.

Cardiology Board Review: ECG, Hemodynamic and Angiographic Unknowns, First Edition. Edited by George A. Stouffer.
© 2019 John Wiley & Sons Ltd. Published 2019 by John Wiley & Sons Ltd.

Ventricular extrasystoles and malignant ventricular arrhythmias such as ventricular tachycardia and ventricular fibrillation can occur with hypokalemia with the risk increased by myocardial ischemia and/or digitalis derivatives. Hypokalemia is an important cause of acquired long QT syndrome (LQTS) and can thus predispose to torsades

Table 27.1 ECG changes associated with electrolyte abnormalities.

	Increased	Decreased
K^+	Tall, narrow, peaked T waves QRS prolongation Decreased amplitude of P waves Absent P waves ST segment elevation in V1 and V2 Sine wave appearance	ST segment depression Decreased T wave amplitude or T wave inversion Prominent U waves (mid precordial leads) QRS widening (children) Arrhythmias and AV block
Ca^+	Decrease in QTc (a short QT interval with minimal ST segment is characteristic of hypercalcemia) No change in morphology of P or T waves PR interval and QRS duration may be prolonged Arrhythmias are uncommon although AV block has been reported Can worsen digitalis toxicity Many patients with hypercalcemia develop hypokalemia	Prolongation of QTc P and T waves usually not affected QRS and PR duration usually not affected
Na^{++}	No effect	No effect
Mg^{++}	Minimal effects; extremely high serum magnesium levels may produce bradycardia or cardiac arrhythmias	Usually minimal effects on the ECG but can co-exist with hypokalemia. Torsades de pointes (multifocal ventricular tachycardia) may be precipitated.

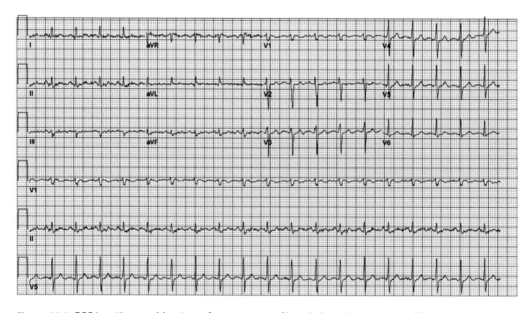

Figure 27.2 ECG in a 42-year-old patient after correction of hypokalemia (K+ = 3.8 mmol/l).

de pointes. Hypokalemia can also cause arrhythmias due to enhanced automaticity.

This patient was hypokalemic (K+ = 2.5 mmol/l) as a result of his illness (causing diarrhea and vomiting) and hydrochlorothiazide. His ECG after correction of his potassium (K+ = 3.8 mmol/l) is shown in Figure 27.2.

Further Reading

Diercks, D.B., Shumaik, G.M., Harrigan, R.A. et al. (2004). Electrocardiographic manifestations: electrolyte abnormalities. *The Journal of Emergency Medicine* 27 (2): 153–160.

El-Sherif, N., & Turitto, G. (2011). Electrolyte disorders and arrhythmogenesis. *Cardiology journal*, 18(3): 233–245.

Case 28: A 58-Year-Old Male with Worsening Dyspnea

You are asked to see a 58-year-old male with past medical history of hypertension and hyperlipidemia who complains of worsening shortness of breath. Symptoms began several weeks ago and have gotten progressively worse. At various times, the dyspnea has been associated with chest pain, dizziness, sweating, and nausea. Prior to the onset of symptoms, the patient had not had any symptoms elicited by exercise or walking.

On physical exam, blood pressure is 118/94 mmHg and heart rate is 91 bpm. The patient has 1+ swelling in both legs, a normal cardiac exam, and mild crackles at both bases on the pulmonary exam.

His laboratory values are significant for a mildly elevated troponin I level (0.073 ng/ml) and markedly elevated NT-pro-BNP (N-terminal pro-B-type natriuretic peptide) level of 5800 pg/ml. ECG is below (Figure 28.1). How do you interpret the BNP (B-type natriuretic peptide) level and what is the mostly likely diagnosis?

Heart Failure

Echocardiography showed poor left ventricular systolic dysfunction, a moderately dilated left ventricle, and diastolic dysfunction. To

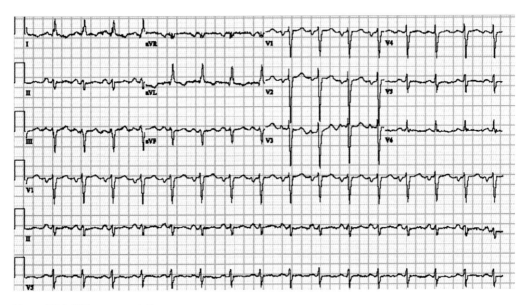

Figure 28.1 ECG on presentation.

Cardiology Board Review: ECG, Hemodynamic and Angiographic Unknowns, First Edition. Edited by George A. Stouffer.
© 2019 John Wiley & Sons Ltd. Published 2019 by John Wiley & Sons Ltd.

further evaluate the cardiomyopathy, the patient undergoes cardiac catheterization which shows no significant coronary artery disease and a left ventricular ejection fraction (LVEF) of 15–20%. The level of elevation of NT-pro-BNP is consistent with heart failure (HF). NT-pro-BNP can also be elevated in acute coronary syndromes (ACS) but rarely exceeds 500 pg/ml and correlates with infarct size. It would be inconsistent in the setting of an ACS to have a pro-BNP level of 5800 pg/ml with only a mildly elevated troponin I level.

There are roughly 650 000 new cases of HF diagnosed each year in the United States with the incidence varying by age: 20 per 1000 in those 65–69 and >80 per 1000 in those older than 84 years (Benjamin et al. 2018). New onset HF can be caused by multiple etiologies, but all primarily lead to the cardinal symptoms of dyspnea, fatigue, and fluid retention, though the exact presentation in each patient can differ widely (Yancy et al. 2013, 2017). While there are various labs and imaging modalities that can suggest new onset HF, it is largely a clinical diagnosis. Beyond the cardinal symptoms, it's important to inquire about gastrointestinal symptoms, weight changes, and palpitations to gauge potential etiologies and severity of disease. It is also important to inquire about current medications and the amount of sodium in the diet. On exam, clues identifying HF can be elicited from orthostatic changes, jugular venous pulse, murmurs, point of maximum impact, pulmonary function, hepatomegaly, and edema (Yancy et al. 2013, 2017; Thibodeau and Drazner 2018).

HF can be classified into HF with reduced EF (HFrEF) or HF with preserved EF (HFpEF), which impacts treatment options and outcomes. HFrEF is defined as a clinical diagnosis of HF and EF ≤ 40% (Yancy et al. 2013). The exact definition of HFpEF varies but generally includes HF signs and symptoms with EF ≥ 50%, with patients with EF in the 40–50% range comprising an intermediate group (Yancy et al. 2013). Proposed criteria for HFpEF include (i) clinical signs or symptoms of HF; (ii) evidence of preserved or normal LVEF; (iii) evidence of abnormal

LV diastolic dysfunction that can be determined by Doppler echocardiography or cardiac catheterization.

The New York Heart Association (NYHA) has four classifications of HF based on symptom severity (Table 28.1). The American College of Cardiology Foundation/American Heart Association (ACCF/AHA) have mapped the progression of HF from stages A through D based on the level of structural damage and symptoms (Table 28.2).

Etiologies of HFrEF include coronary artery disease, diabetes, hypertension, alcohol, obesity, familial cardiomyopathies, thyroid disease, acromegaly, tachycardia-induced cardiomyopathy, cocaine use, myocarditis, acquired immunodeficiency syndrome, chemotherapy,

Table 28.1 New York Heart Association Functional Classification.

Class	Functional Classification
I	No limitation of physical activity. Ordinary physical activity does not cause symptoms of HF.
II	Slight limitation of physical activity. Comfortable at rest, but ordinary physical activity results in symptoms of HF.
III	Marked limitation of physical activity. Comfortable at rest, but less than ordinary activity causes symptoms of HF.
IV	Unable to carry on any physical activity without symptoms of HF, or symptoms of HF at rest.

Table 28.2 American College of Cardiology Foundation/American Heart Association (ACCF/AHA) stages of HF.

Stage	
A	At high risk for HF but without structural heart disease or symptoms of HF.
B	Structural heart disease but without signs or symptoms of HF.
C	Structural heart disease with prior or current symptoms of HF.
D	Refractory HF requiring specialized interventions

Source: Modified from Yancy et al. (2013).

peripartum cardiomyopathy, hemochromatosis, Takotsubo (stress-induced cardiomyopathy), amyloidosis, cardiac sarcoidosis, and valvular heart disease. Many of the same etiologies can cause diastolic dysfunction with the most common being ischemic heart disease, hypertrophic obstructive cardiomyopathy, and restrictive heart disease.

Use of Natriuretic Peptide Biomarkers in the Diagnosis and Management of HF

There are two natriuretic peptides used in the diagnosis and management of HF – BNP and NT-pro-BNP. Both natriuretic peptide biomarker values track together and either can be used in patient care settings. Their respective absolute values and cutpoints are different and they cannot be used interchangeably in the same patient. The production of BNP and NT-pro-BNP involves a process initiated by myocyte stretch resulting in the production of pre-pro-BNP which undergoes cleavage into measurable BNP and NT-pro-BNP (Maisel et al. 2018). One significant difference is that BNP, but not NT-pro-BNP, is a substrate for neprilysin. Therefore, angiotensin receptor-neprilysin inhibition increases BNP levels but not NT-pro-BNP levels.

While HF is largely diagnosed based on patient history and clinical presentation, with particular emphasis on volume status, a number of laboratory and diagnostic tests, especially natriuretic peptides, are available to support a diagnosis of HF and classify it as HFrEF or HFpEF (Yancy et al. 2017). Low BNP or NT-pro-BNP levels can be informative to exclude a diagnosis of HF as they have high negative predictive values; a BNP <100 pg/ml and a NT-pro-BNP <300 pg/ml have a negative predictive value of 98% for the diagnosis of HF (Maisel et al. 2018). Typically, patients in HF have BNP > 400 pg/ml or NT-pro-BNP >450, 900, and 1800 pg/ml for patients <50, 50–75, and >75 years old, respectively (Francis et al. 2016; Chang et al. 2017; Maisel et al. 2018). These initial tests and lab values enable proper classification and help decide a proper treatment regime.

Particularly with HFpEF, it is important to consider that a patient's symptoms can be a result of other conditions – obesity, lung disease, coronary ischemia – that may present similarly to HF (Yancy et al. 2017). While BNP or NT-pro-BNP levels are useful in excluding the diagnosis of HF, there are other conditions that can cause increased levels. Some of these include coronary artery disease, renal dysfunction, pulmonary embolism, valvular heart disease, hypertension, and lung disease, among others; therefore, it's important to take into account a patient's clinical presentation (Yancy et al. 2017).

BNP and NT-pro-BNP levels provide useful information beyond initial diagnosis of HF; they can be utilized to guide therapy and for prognostic purposes. Serial measurements of natriuretic peptide during hospitalization can be beneficial as levels are expected to decrease. Consistently high levels or baseline levels, BNP > 200 pg/ml or NT-pro-BNP >986 pg/ml, are associated with worse prognosis (Maisel et al. 2018). A meta-analysis showed that there is a 35% increased risk of death for every 100 pg/ml increase in BNP level (Doust et al. 2005). There are promising data showing the benefit of serial measurements, and it is a widely adopted clinical practice. The class of recommendation and level of evidence is 1 and A, respectively, for utilizing natriuretic peptides levels for management of and prognosis in HF (Yancy et al. 2013, 2017).

References

Benjamin, E.J., Virani, S.S., Callaway, C.W. et al. (2018). Heart disease and stroke Statistics-2018 update: a report from the American Heart Association. *Circulation* 137 (12): e67–e492. https://doi.org/10.1161/CIR.0000000000000558. Epub 2018 Jan 31.

Chang, K.W., Fox, S., Mojaver, S. et al. (2017). Using biomarkers to guide heart failure management. *Expert Review of Cardiovascular Therapy* 15 (10): 729–741. https://doi.org/10.1080/14779072.2017. 1366312. Epub 2017 Aug 22.

Doust, J.A., Pietrzak, E., Dobson, A. et al. (2005). How well does B-type natriuretic peptide predict death and cardiac events in patients with heart failure: systematic review. *BMJ* 330 (7492): 625. https://doi. org/10.1136/bmj.330.7492.625.

Francis, G.S., Felker, G.M., and Tang, W.H. (2016). A test in context: critical evaluation of natriuretic peptide testing in heart failure. *Journal of the American College of Cardiology* 67 (3): 330–337. https://doi. org/10.1016/j.jacc.2015.10.073.

Maisel, A.S., Duran, J.M., and Wettersten, N. (2018). Natriuretic peptides in heart failure: atrial and B-type natriuretic peptides. *Heart Failure Clinics* 14 (1): 13–25. https://doi. org/10.1016/j.hfc.2017.08.002.

Thibodeau, J.T. and Drazner, M.H. (2018). The role of the clinical examination in patients with heart failure. *JACC Heart Fail* 31 (18): 005.

Yancy, C.W., Jessup, M., Bozkurt, B. et al. (2013). 2013 ACCF/AHA guideline for the management of heart failure: a report of the American College of Cardiology Foundation/American Heart Association Task Force on Practice Guidelines. *Journal of the American College of Cardiology* 62 (16): e147–e239. https://doi.org/10.1016/j. jacc.2013.05.019. Epub 2013 Jun 5.

Yancy, C.W., Jessup, M., Bozkurt, B. et al. (2017). 2017 ACC/AHA/HFSA focused update of the 2013 ACCF/AHA guideline for the Management of Heart Failure: a report of the American College of Cardiology/American Heart Association Task Force on Clinical Practice Guidelines and the Heart Failure Society of America. *Journal of the American College of Cardiology* 70 (6): 776–803. https://doi. org/10.1016/j.jacc.2017.04.025. Epub 2017 Apr 28.

Case 29: A 68-Year-Old Woman with Chest Pain and a Normal Stress Test

A 68-year-old female presented to her primary care physician (PCP) with complaints of chest tightness while riding her stationary bike. The symptoms reliably occurred after 10 minutes of exercise and got better when she stopped bicycling. She had no known coronary artery disease but did have hypercholesterolemia, hypertension, insulin-dependent diabetes, chronic kidney disease (baseline creatinine 2.15 mg/dl, glomerular filtration rate 23 ml/min/1.73 m^2), previous ischemic stroke without residual deficits, and ongoing tobacco abuse with moderate to severe chronic obstructive pulmonary disease (COPD). Her PCP ordered a single-photon emission computed tomography (SPECT) nuclear stress test which did not show any focal perfusion defects and a transthoracic echocardiogram (TTE) which was notable for normal ejection fraction and no significant valvular disease.

When her symptoms persisted, the PCP sent the patient to you for further evaluation. Her ECG is below (Figure 29.1). What is the next step in the diagnostic workup?

Additional Evaluation

The next step in the diagnostic evaluation is to recommend coronary angiography. The patient had multiple risk factors (diabetes,

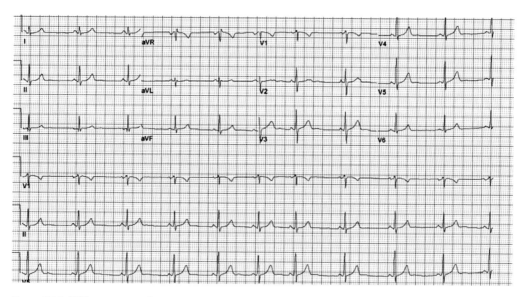

Figure 29.1 ECG on presentation.

Cardiology Board Review: ECG, Hemodynamic and Angiographic Unknowns, First Edition. Edited by George A. Stouffer.
© 2019 John Wiley & Sons Ltd. Published 2019 by John Wiley & Sons Ltd.

hypertension, hyperlipidemia, tobacco use, and chronic kidney disease) and typical sounding angina (exertional angina relieved by rest). As illustrated by Diamond and Forrester in their classic article outlining the use of Bayesian probability in the diagnosis of coronary artery disease (CAD), the poststress test probability of CAD depends on pretest probability and results of the stress test (Diamond and Forrester 1979). They found that the prevalence of obstructive CAD was 90% in females between the ages of 60 and 69 with typical symptoms. The likelihood of CAD was even greater when risk factors were taken into consideration. A negative stress test lowers the probability but it still remains >70% that the patient has obstructive CAD. A normal ECG (as in this patient) does not preclude severe coronary artery disease.

Coronary angiography revealed a severe, 90% non-calcified left main coronary artery (LMCA) lesion primarily involving the mid to distal segment of a long left main artery (Figure 29.2). Angiography performed after intracoronary nitroglycerin did not show any improvement in the stenosis. The right coronary artery (RCA) was a dominant vessel with mild, nonobstructive plaque in the mid artery.

Treatment

Based on her anatomy, the Synergy Between Percutaneous Coronary Intervention With Taxus and Cardiac Surgery (SYNTAX) score describing her disease was 11 (Kappetein et al. 2006). Incorporating her clinical and comorbid conditions, the SYNTAX II score was 45.7 for percutaneous coronary intervention (PCI) and 44.9 for coronary artery bypass grafting (CABG) (Farooq et al. 2013). Given the severity of stenosis, the patient's preference to avoid CABG, and her underlying pulmonary disease, the decision was made to treat the LMCA lesion percutaneously. Using intravascular ultrasound (IVUS) guidance, a drug-eluting stent was deployed in the left main (Figure 29.3). The patient recovered well and her angina resolved. Renal function

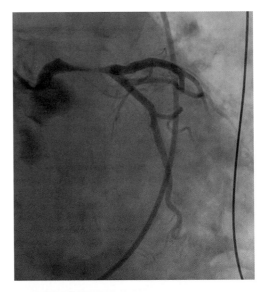

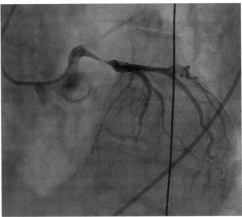

Figure 29.2 Coronary angiography in AP (anteroposterior) caudal and LAO (left anterior oblique) cranial views showing a severe 90% non-calcified left main lesion primarily involving the mid to distal left main.

remained stable. Aggressive secondary medical prevention was initiated including risk factor modification and smoking cessation.

Disease of the Left Main Coronary Artery

This patient presented with unsuspected left main disease with classic progressive angina symptoms but a normal nuclear perfusion

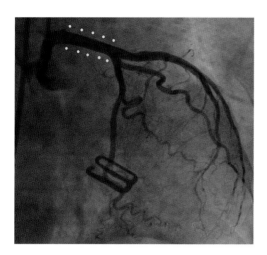

Figure 29.3 Coronary angiography showing successful percutaneous coronary intervention (PCI) with a drug-eluting stent. Stent length outlined in yellow.

stress test. Although rare, SPECT nuclear stress tests can yield a false negative result in the setting of multivessel coronary disease or left main disease due to relatively "balanced" ischemia. The prevalence of false negative SPECT results was found to approach 7% in a population at high risk for CAD in an article by Nakanishi and colleagues (Nakanishi et al. 2016). In a population with a high pretest probability of CAD, such as our patient presenting with classic and concerning progressive angina with multiple CAD risk factors, there should be a high index of suspicion for obstructive CAD.

Revascularization

Decisions about revascularization for left main coronary disease have evolved as PCI techniques have improved. Given the poor natural history of purely medically managed left main disease seen in early revascularization trials evaluating CABG versus medical therapy (although it is important to note that medical management is now much better than it was during those trials), current guidelines recommend revascularization of left main disease >50%, regardless of symptom status (Chaitman et al. 1981; Yusuf et al. 1994; Levine et al. 2011). Revascularization can be

done by CABG or PCI. Deciding which modality to use relies on the characteristics of disease including location (ostial, mid, or distal) and presence or absence of calcification. In addition, the presence of other obstructive concomitant epicardial coronary artery disease, the patient's operative risk, and patient preference are major factors in deciding the method of revascularization.

Coronary Artery Bypass Grafting or Percutaneous Coronary Intervention

Early revascularization trials focused on CABG versus medical therapy showed a mortality benefit in favor of CABG, particularly when using a left internal mammary artery to LAD (left anterior descending) bypass graft (Yusuf et al. 1994). More contemporary randomized control trials have compared PCI and CABG in patients with LMCA disease. The SYNTAX trial compared outcomes between PCI with a paclitaxel-eluting first-generation drug-eluting stent and CABG in patients with multivessel disease (Mohr et al. 2013). A SYNTAX score encompassing angiographic findings to quantify the complexity of disease was developed and validated to stratify the different patients enrolled. Based on the five-year results, the LMCA substudy of the SYNTAX trial showed that PCI was noninferior to CABG in regards to death and myocardial infarction (MI) across the spectrum of SYNTAX scores. CABG was superior to PCI at five years in terms of repeat revascularization in the more complex disease cohort (SYNTAX score > 32). The rate of stroke was increased in the CABG cohort.

The SYNTAX score is an angiography-based tool derived from the summation of the individual scores for each separate lesion with ≥50% luminal obstruction in vessels ≥1.5 mm. It quantitatively characterizes the coronary vasculature with respect to the number, location, complexity, and functional impact of angiographically obstructive lesions. Important anatomic factors include diffuse disease, thrombus, calcification, tortuosity, total occlusions, bi- and trifurcations, aorto-ostial location, length, and dominance. The distributions of the coronary arteries are mapped based on the ARTS (Arterial Revascularization Therapies Study) and each coronary segment is weighted according to the fraction of blood supplied to the left ventricle. SYNTAX scores are generally divided into tertiles as low: 0–22, intermediate: 23–32, and high: >32.

Current guidelines list PCI of LMCA disease as a 2a recommendation for mid shaft and ostial disease in the absence of significant other major epicardial CAD stenosis and assuming surgical risk is high. Based on results of the SYNTAX trial, it is a 2b recommendation for left main PCI in the setting of other coronary disease if the overall SYNTAX score <32 and surgical risk is high. It is a class 3 recommendation to perform LMCA PCI in the setting of other multivessel CAD and SYNTAX score >32 in a good surgical candidate (Levine et al. 2011). Critiques of the SYNTAX trial include the lack of physiological data to supplement angiographic findings and use of paclitaxel-coated stents.

Newer drug-eluting stents have shown reduced rates of target vessel revascularization and stent thrombosis compared to paclitaxel-eluting stents (Alazzoni et al. 2012). To reflect current practice, two more contemporary trials: EXCEL (Evaluation of XIENCE versus Coronary Artery Bypass Surgery for Effectiveness of Left Main Revascularization) and NOBLE (the Nordic-Baltic-British Left Main Revascularization Study) were conducted to compare PCI and CABG outcomes for LMCA disease (Mäkikallio et al. 2016; Stone et al. 2016). For both of these trials, patients had a low prevalence of diabetes and left ventricular ejection fraction (LVEF) was preserved. The average SYNTAX score ranged between 22 and 26. Roughly 75% of LMCA PCIs were optimized with IVUS in these trials. In both EXCEL and NOBLE, PCI was noninferior to CABG at three years of follow up in regards to death and stroke. In EXCEL, PCI was noninferior to CABG for MI but had increased rates of repeat revascularization. For NOBLE, PCI had increased rates of MI and repeat revascularization. Neither of these

trials are currently reflected in current US guidelines. Understanding which patient subgroups benefit more from either modality needs to be a key focus of future research. Best practice guidelines recommend using a heart team approach to evaluate patients prior to left main revascularization. This approach should encompass traditional risk models such as the STS score and SYNTAX. In addition, other variables not easily captured in traditional models, such as frailty and patient preference, should be factored into revascularization decisions.

In our patient, the left main disease was mostly confined to the mid vessel and spared the true distal left main bifurcation. Given her low SYNTAX score, this was an acceptable lesion for PCI. In addition, the Syntax II score was equivalent for PCI and CABG (Farooq 2013). According to the latest guidelines, PCI for ostial or mid-shaft left main lesions in the setting of SYNTAX score <22 and with estimated CABG mortality >5% is a class 2a recommendation (Levine et al. 2011). For our patient, using the Society of Thoracic Surgeons (STS) Adult Cardiac Surgery Database Version 2.81 risk calculator, the estimated risk of mortality with CABG was 5.1% (STS Adult Cardiac Surgery Risk Calculator. Database Version 2.81. Online: http://riskcalc.sts.org). Her intervention was performed using IVUS guidance and without mechanical hemodynamic support.

Intravascular Ultrasound in Left Main Disease

IVUS has been validated as an important tool for determining left main severity in cases where angiography is unclear regarding disease severity. IVUS can also help in determining the location and composition of left main disease and can help optimize stent sizing and deployment. de la Torre Hernandez and colleagues helped validate IVUS in the LMCA prospectively using a cutoff luminal area to determine safety for deferring revascularization for LMCA disease (de la Torre Hernandez et al. 2011, 2007). Based on their research, deferring intervention in the scenario of stable angina and LMCA minimal luminal area (MLA) > 6 mm^2 was noted to be as efficacious as undergoing intervention. Importantly, there was a signal that patients with MLA between 5 and 6 mm^2 and who deferred intervention had worse outcomes. Also highlighted by de la Torre Hernandez was the limitation of angiography to determine severity as a third of patients with angiographic stenosis <30% also by IVUS had a MLA < 6 mm^2. Conversely, 43% of patients with a stenosis >50% had a MLA > 6 mm^2, which they showed can be safely deferred.

There are problems with using a hard cutoff for all patients, as there is notable ethnic variability in normal LMCA MLA. Rusinova et al. showed that in a stable cohort of Asian and Caucasian patients, the LMCA MLA is smaller in Asians (5.2 ± 1.8 vs 6.2 ± 14 mm^2; $P < 0.0001$) (Rusinova et al. 2013). Therefore, a physiologic assessment of LMCA disease severity is important in ambiguous stenosis severity. IVUS has also been shown to improve rates of cardiac death, myocardial infarction, and target lesion revascularization at three years when used to optimize PCI results (de la Torre Hernandez et al. 2014).

Fractional Flow Reserve

In 2004, Vanu Jasti and colleagues showed that a MLA from IVUS of >5.9 mm^2 correlated with a fractional flow reserve (FFR) value of >0.75 (Jasti et al. 2004). A more recent Korean study instead found that an IVUS MLA cutoff of 4.5 mm^2 correlated with an FFR value of 0.80 (Park et al. 2014). This variability again highlights ethnic differences in normal LMCA size and also the importance of knowing the physiologic significance of ambiguous disease to help best determine safety of deferring revascularization. Hamilos and colleagues were able to show LMCA lesions were able to be safely deferred for FFR values >0.80 (Hamilos et al. 2009). As with IVUS, there was a wide range of variability of angiography assessment of disease severity above a FFR of 0.80.

Future clinical outcomes trials are needed to support the use of instantaneous wave-free ratio (iFR) to guide revascularization decisions. Optical coherence tomography (OCT) is less widely used to visualize LMCA disease, as displacement of blood by contrast to obtain quality images can be technically challenging.

References

Alazzoni, A., Al-Saleh, A., and Jolly, S.S. (2012). Everolimus-eluting versus paclitaxel-eluting stents in percutaneous coronary intervention: meta-analysis of randomized trials. *Thrombosis* 2012: 126369. https://doi.org/10.1155/2012/126369.

Chaitman, B.R., Fisher, L.D., Bourassa, M.G. et al. (1981). Effect of coronary bypass surgery on survival patterns in subsets of patients with left main coronary artery disease: report of the Collaborative Study in Coronary Artery Surgery (CASS). *The American Journal of Cardiology* 48 (4): 765–777.

Diamond, G.A. and Forrester, J.S. (1979). Analysis of probability as an aid in the clinical diagnosis of coronary-artery disease. *New England Journal of Medicine* 300 (24): 1350–1358.

Farooq, V., Van Klaveren, D., Steyerberg, E.W. et al. (2013). Anatomical and clinical characteristics to guide decision making between coronary artery bypass surgery and percutaneous coronary intervention for individual patients: development and validation of SYNTAX score II. *Lancet* 381 (9867): 639–650.

Hamilos, M., Muller, O., Cuisset, T. et al. (2009). Long-term clinical outcome after fractional flow reserve-guided treatment in patients with angiographically equivocal left main coronary artery stenosis. *Circulation* 120 (15): 1505–1512.

Jasti, V., Ivan, E., Yalamanchili, V. et al. (2004). Correlations between fractional flow reserve and intravascular ultrasound in patients with an ambiguous left main coronary artery stenosis. *Circulation* 110 (18): 2831–2836.

Kappetein, A.P., Dawkins, K.D., Mohr, F.W. et al. (2006). Current percutaneous coronary intervention and coronary artery bypass grafting practices for three-vessel and left main coronary artery disease. Insights from the SYNTAX run-in phase. *European Journal of Cardio-Thoracic Surgery* 29: 486–491.

Levine, G.N., Bates, E.R., Blankenship, J.C. et al. (2011). 2011 ACCF/AHA/SCAI guideline for percutaneous coronary intervention. A report of the American College of Cardiology Foundation/American Heart Association task force on practice guidelines and the Society for Cardiovascular Angiography and Interventions. *Journal of the American College of Cardiology* 58: e44–e122.

Mäkikallio, T., Holm, N.R., Lindsay, M. et al. (2016). Percutaneous coronary angioplasty versus coronary artery bypass grafting in treatment of unprotected left main stenosis (NOBLE): a prospective, randomised, open-label, non-inferiority trial. *Lancet* 388: 2743–2752.

Mohr, F., Morice, M.C., Kappetein, A.P. et al. (2013). Coronary artery bypass graft surgery versus percutaneous coronary intervention in patients with three-vessel disease and left main coronary disease: 5-year follow-up of the randomised, clinical SYNTAX trial. *Lancet* 381: 629–638.

Nakanishi, R., Gransar, H., Slomka, P. et al. (2016). Predictors of high risk coronary artery disease in subjects with normal SPECT myocardial perfusion imaging. *Journal of Nuclear Cardiology* 23 (3): 530–541.

Park, S.J., Ahn, J.M., Kang, S.J. et al. (2014). Intravascular ultrasound-derived minimal lumen area criteria for functionally significant left main coronary artery stenosis. *JACC Cardiovascular Interventions* 7 (8): 868–874.

Rusinova, R.P., Mintz, G.S., Choi, S.Y. et al. (2013). Intravascular ultrasound comparison of left main coronary artery disease between white and Asian patients. *The American Journal of Cardiology* 111 (7): 979–984.

Stone, G.W., Sabik, J.F., Serruys, P.W. et al. (2016). Everolimus-eluting stents or bypass surgery for left main coronary artery disease. *The New England Journal of Medicine* 375: 2223–2235.

de la Torre Hernandez, J.M., Alfonso, F.M., Garcia, T.C. et al. (2014). Clinical impact of intravascular ultrasound guidance in drug-eluting stent implantation for unprotected left main coronary disease: pooled analysis at the patient-level of 4 registries. *JACC Cardiovascular Interventions* 7 (3): 244–254.

de la Torre Hernandez, J.M., Hernández Hernandez, F., Alfonso, F. et al. (2011). Prospective application of pre-defined intravascular ultrasound criteria for assessment of intermediate left main coronary artery lesions results from the multicenter LITRO study. *Journal of the American College of Cardiology* 58 (4): 351–358.

de la Torre Hernandez, J.M., Ruiz Lera, M., Fernandez Friera, L. et al. (2007). Prospective use of an intravascular ultrasound-derived minimum lumen area cut-off value in the assessment of intermediate left main coronary artery lesions. *Revista Española de Cardiología* 60: 811–816.

Yusuf, S., Zucker, D., Passamani, E. et al. (1994). Effect of coronary artery bypass graft surgery on survival: overview of 10-year results from randomised trials by the Coronary Artery Bypass Graft Surgery Trialists Collaboration. *Lancet* 344: 563–570.

Case 30: A 29-Year-Old Woman with Shortness of Breath and Leg Swelling

A 29-year-old woman without significant medical history is referred to you for evaluation of shortness of breath and leg swelling. When she was in high school she participated on the swimming team and has since continued to swim three to four times a week for exercise. However, she began noticing her exertional capacity diminishing one year ago and in the last three months, she has not been able to swim at all. Additionally, she reports a sense of abdominal fullness and ankle swelling which she finds very concerning.

Physical examination reveals a generally well-appearing woman in no acute distress. On auscultation, aortic and pulmonic components of the second heart sound remain split during both inspiration and expiration. A soft II/VI holosystolic murmur that varies with respiration is heard at the left lower sternal border. She has hepatomegaly on abdominal exam and mild pedal edema bilaterally. Neck findings include giant "cv" waves up to her mandible. Laboratory panel shows normal complete blood count, metabolic panel, and thyroid function. Electrocardiogram reveals an incomplete right bundle branch block (RBBB) with R wave notches in leads II, III, and aVF (Figure 30.1).

What is the most likely diagnosis and the next diagnostic step?

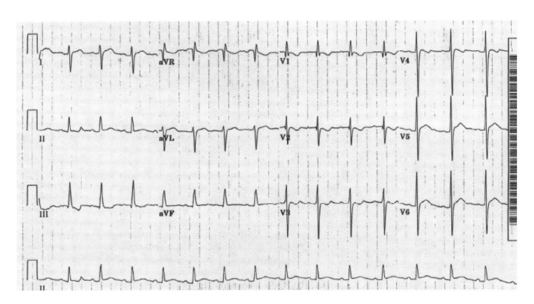

Figure 30.1 ECG in a 29-year-old female with shortness of breath.

Cardiology Board Review: ECG, Hemodynamic and Angiographic Unknowns, First Edition. Edited by George A. Stouffer.
© 2019 John Wiley & Sons Ltd. Published 2019 by John Wiley & Sons Ltd.

Ostium Secundum Atrial Septal Defect

The ECG and examination are consistent with a secundum atrial septal defect (ASD), a congenital defect creating an opening in the septum between the two atria at the fossa ovalis and ostium secundum. This defect usually arises because the septum secundum cannot cover a large ostium secundum due to increased resorption; it can also be caused by inadequate formation of the septum secundum.

Common physical exam findings in patients with ostium secundum ASD include fixed split S2 and a systolic murmur heard best at the left upper sternal border. This murmur reflects increased flow across the pulmonary valve. There is no murmur associated with flow across an ostium secundum ASD. A loud P2 is occasionally present and suggests pulmonary hypertension.

The most characteristic ECG finding in patients with an ostium secundum ASD is an rSR′ or rSr′ pattern in lead V1 with a QRS duration of less than 110 ms. This finding is observed in approximately 60% of patients with an ASD. Complete RBBB is found in 5–19% of ASD cases, but less prevalently in younger patients such as this one. The mean QRS axis is usually greater than 100°, and almost always between 0 and 180° in secundum type ASD. Voltage evidence of right ventricular hypertrophy (RVH) may be seen in ASDs and becomes more pronounced as pulmonary hypertension progresses. In most patients, P wave morphology is normal although right atrial enlargement can be present.

This ECG shows a pronounced R wave in lead V1, marked right axis deviation, and evidence of RVH. These findings suggest right heart pathology and warrant further investigation. Echocardiography showed the presence of a moderate size secundum ASD with significant left-to-right shunting on color Doppler flow imaging (Figure 30.2). The right ventricle is severely dilated with associated severe tricuspid regurgitation. Quantitative assessment with cardiac MRI (magnetic resonance imaging) confirms her severely dilated right ventricle and shows a Qp/Qs of 3 : 1 (Figure 30.3).

Case Summary

This patient's constellation of symptoms, physical exam findings, and clinical tests are representative of a large, unrestricted

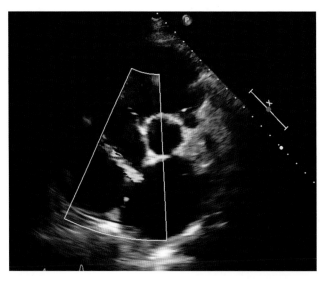

Figure 30.2 Transthoracic echocardiography short axis view showing presence of moderate size secundum atrial septal defect with significant left-to-right shunting on color Doppler flow imaging.

secundum ASD with ensuing development of right heart failure. Her relatively healthy status as a young adult suggests a nonsignificant shunt during adolescence allowing adequate exertional capacity and ultimately leading to a delayed presentation. Fixed splitting of the S2 is a staple of ASD and the associated holosystolic murmur with jugular vein findings is representative of severe tricuspid regurgitation, ostensibly secondary to right heart dilation and failure. An assessment of right- and left-sided cardiac output (Qp and Qs) in this case helps to quantify the extent of left-to-right shunting.

Clinical Presentation of ASD

ASD is the most common congenital cardiac abnormality in adults in the United States. There are four types of ASDs: ostium primum, ostium secundum, sinus venosus, and coronary sinus defects (Figure 30.4). Secundum defects are the most common, comprising just over 70% of all ASDs. Most secundum ASDs do not have any consequences during childhood and adolescence, with most pathologic manifestations occurring in adulthood. Clinical presentation includes arrhythmias, stroke due to paradoxical embolism, as well as right-sided heart failure and pulmonary hypertension.

Since left-sided cardiac chamber pressures are higher than right-sided pressures, the presence of a direct communication between the left atrium and right atrium leads initially to left-to-right shunting (in the absence of a Valsalva maneuver). In a small ASD (<5 mm), this shunting may be clinically insignificant. However, moderate-to-large ASDs can result in more substantial left-to-right shunting resulting in right ventricular volume overload, right ventricular dilation, and right atrial enlargement. Patients can develop pulmonary hypertension (with histopathological changes of endothelial dysfunction and vascular remodeling with proliferative changes) and atrial arrhythmias secondary to atrial stretch and fibrosis. They may also complain of shortness of breath as well as other signs of right heart failure – fluid retention, hepatosplenomegaly, and elevated jugular venous distension. If this condition remains uncorrected, pulmonary artery pressures can dramatically rise, leading to suprasystemic levels and finally result in right-to-left shunting (known as Eisenmenger's syndrome).

The presence of a secundum ASD also creates an anatomical condition in which venous thrombi can cross over from the venous to arterial circulation and consequently result in stroke, transient ischemic attack, or other arterial embolism (termed *paradoxical embolism)*. Paradoxical emboli are relatively rare but represent a clinically significant sequela of ASD and may be the first clinical presentation in this cohort of patients.

Pathophysiology

During normal embryologic development, the atrial septum is formed by the caudal growth of the septum primum from the superior aspect of the atrium until it reaches the endocardial cushions. The ostium secundum then forms within the central portion of the newly formed septum primum. The septum secundum is a second growth which grows caudally on the right atrial aspect of the septum primum and then generally covers the ostium secundum. After birth, there is commonly fusion of the septum primum and septum secundum with formation of the fossa ovalis at the location of the ostium secundum overlap. In circumstances where the septum secundum growth does not cover the septum primum, the residual communication between the left and right atria is termed a secundum ASD. The clinical presentation and subsequent clinical ramifications of ASD depend largely on the size and extent of shunting.

Diagnosis

Secundum ASDs are frequently not detected by fetal echocardiography. As patients are not usually symptomatic in childhood, particularly in small ASDs, presentation during adulthood is common. On physical examination, a widely, fixed split second heart sound may be observed. During normal physiology, inspiration leads to increased right-sided cardiac filling with resulting delayed closure of the pulmonic valve and a split second heart sound. This effect disappears with expiration as the aortic and pulmonic valves close at relatively the same time. In the presence of a left-to-right shunt with secundum ASD, S2 remains split as during expiration, blood flow from the left heart results in increased right ventricular filling and once again delays the closure of the pulmonic valve.

In addition to physical examination, comprehensive echocardiography is a mainstay in the diagnosis of secundum ASDs. In addition to visualization of the defect, transthoracic echocardiography can be helpful in quantifying pulmonary artery pressures and estimating shunt magnitude. Transesophageal echocardiography is a useful adjunct to measure septal defect margins in multiple dimensions and allow for planning of either percutaneous or surgical ASD closure. MRI is not required for the evaluation of all ASDs but can be used to further quantify shunt severity; the use of cardiac MRI is most helpful in those circumstances in which echocardiography cannot conclusively demonstrate

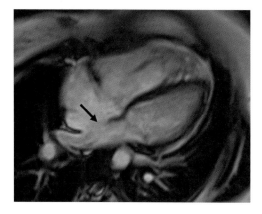

Figure 30.3 Cardiac MRI shows presence of secundum atrial septal defect (arrow) with dilated right atrium and right ventricle (upper most ventricle in this image).

pathology but clinical index of suspicion is high. The most recent ACC/AHA (American College of Cardiologists/American Heart Association) guidelines for the diagnosis of ASDs have a class 1 indication for an imaging technique to diagnose ASD and/or refer to a center with the capability to do so in those patients with unexplained right ventricular volume overload.

Management

Many small ASDs close spontaneously and do not require further evaluation. In patients with moderate-to-large ASDs, correction of shunting may become necessary due to risk of development of right heart failure as well as pulmonary hypertension. Correction can be done either surgically or percutaneously. Most but not all secundum ASDs are candidates for percutaneous closure – i.e. a defect ≤38 mm in diameter with a rim of tissue >5 mm around the defect with the anatomy such that there is a minimal risk of obstructing the coronary sinus, right pulmonary veins, vena cavae, or atrioventricular valves. The most frequently implanted devices when done percutaneously consist of fabric mesh covering opposable double discs, a helix spiral occluder, or two square umbrella-like spring frames. Surgical closure is usually done using pericardium or Dacron and is generally reserved for those patients in whom percutaneous repair is not feasible or appropriate.

Secundum ASD closure (either percutaneously or surgically) is indicated for asymptomatic patients with right atrial or right ventricular enlargement (class 1). Surgical closure of a secundum ASD is reasonable when concomitant surgical repair or replacement of the tricuspid valve is considered, or if percutaneous therapy cannot be offered due to anatomical reasons (class 2a). ASD closure is also reasonable in patients who present with paradoxical embolism (2a). ASD closure is contraindicated in patients with severe, irreversible pulmonary arterial hypertension and no evidence of left-to-right shunt (class 3). During follow-up visits, the patient should be evaluated for development of new arrhythmias and pulmonary pressures, right ventricular function, and residual shunting should be assessed. Additionally, in those patients who develop atrial fibrillation as a consequence of an ASD, cardioversion after appropriate anticoagulation is recommended to restore sinus rhythm; rate control and anticoagulation is recommended if rhythm control cannot be achieved (class 1).

Differentiation of Primum and Secundum ASD

ASDs occur in four locations: ostium secundum, ostium primum, sinus venosus and coronary sinus (Figure 30.4). The ostium secundum is the most common form of ASD and is a true defect of the atrial septum involving the region of the fossa ovalis. The most common associated cardiac anomaly associated with a secundum ASD is a persistent left superior vena cava (SVC) draining

into the coronary sinus. Ostium primum defects are more extensive (also known as AV canal defects or endocardial cushion defects) and usually involve the tricuspid and mitral valves. The complete form of this defect includes a ventricular septal defect and a common atrioventricular valve. Ostium primum defects are present in approximately 15% of patients with Down Syndrome. Sinus venosus defects are usually located at the junction of the right atrium and superior vena cava and are commonly associated with partial anomalous pulmonary venous return. Rarely, sinus venosus defects can involve the inferior vena cava. Another rare type of ASD involves a defect between the coronary sinus and the left atrium.

Frontal plane QRS axis is the most important indicator for differentiation between primum and secundum type ASD. Most patients with primum type ASD have left axis deviation beyond −30°. Right axis deviation between −90 and −180 is so rare in ostium primum ASD as to call the diagnosis into question. First-degree heart block suggests a primum ASD but may be seen in older patients with a secundum ASD.

Case Resolution

The 29-year-old patient underwent transesophageal echocardiography to better characterize the anatomy of the secundum ASD. Adequate septal margins were identified and the patient underwent percutaneous ASD closure with placement of an Amplatzer occluding device. During post-procedure follow-up, she had improved exertional capacity and echocardiogram showed decreased right ventricular size and improved function.

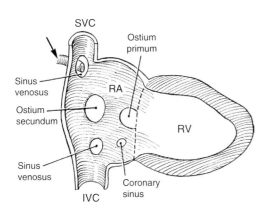

Figure 30.4 Different types of atrial septal defects (IVC = inferior vena cava and SVC = superior vena cava).

Further Reading

Bannan, A., Shen, R., Silvestry, F.E. et al. (2009). Characteristics of adult patients with atrial septal defects presenting with paradoxical embolism. *Catheterization and Cardiovascular Interventions* 74 (7): 1066–1069.

Bhattacharyya, P.J. (2016). 'Crochetage' sign on ECG in secundum ASD: clinical significance. *BMJ Case Reports* 8: 2016.

Hanslik, A., Pospisil, U., Salzer-Muhar, U. et al. (2006). Predictors of spontaneous closure of isolated secundum atrial septal defect in children: a longitudinal study. *Pediatrics* 118 (4): 1560–1565.

Helgason, H. and Jonsdottir, G. (1999). Spontaneous closure of atrial septal defects. *Pediatric Cardiology* 20 (3): 195–199.

O'byrne, M.L., Glatz, A.C., and Gillespie, M.J. (2018). Transcatheter device closure of atrial septal defects: more to think about than just closing the hole. *Current Opinion in Cardiology* 33 (1): 108–116.

Rigatelli, G., Dell'avvocata, F., Tarantini, G. et al. (2014). Clinical, hemodynamic, and intracardiac echocardiographic characteristics of secundum atrial septal defects-related paradoxical embolism in adulthood. *Journal of Interventional Cardiology* 27 (6): 542–547.

Stout, K.K., Daniels, C.J., Aboulhosn, J.A. et al. (2018 Aug 10). 2018 AHA/ACC guideline for the Management of Adults with Congenital Heart Disease: a report of the American College of Cardiology/American Heart Association Task Force on Clinical Practice Guidelines. *Journal of the American College of Cardiology* pii: S0735-1097(18)36845-1. https://doi.org/10.1016/j.jacc.2018.08.1028.

Van der Linde, D., Konings, E.E., Slager, M.A. et al. (2011). Birth prevalence of congenital heart disease worldwide: a systematic review and meta-analysis. *Journal of the American College of Cardiology* 58: 2241–2247.

Case 31: An ECG Finding You Don't Want to Miss

A 31-year-old healthy female is referred to your office for a pre-employment physical. She feels well and has no complaints. She is a nonsmoker and her family history is unremarkable but limited since her father died in an automobile accident at age 35. Physical examination reveals a well appearing female with normal vital signs and normal cardio-vascular examination.

The following ECG is obtained (Figure 31.1). What is the diagnosis?

Long QT Syndrome

This patient has long QT syndrome (LQTS), a genetic disorder that is associated with polymorphous ventricular tachycardia (torsades de pointes) causing syncope and sudden cardiac death.

The QT interval represents the time from the onset of ventricular activation to the end of ventricular repolarization and is thus measured from the beginning of the QRS

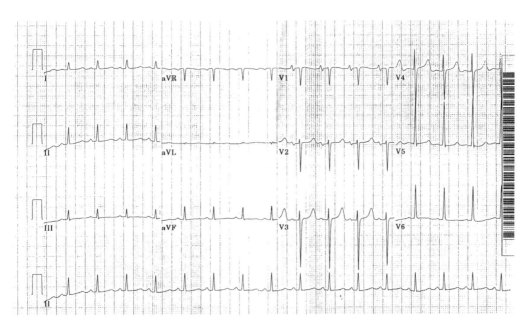

Figure 31.1 ECG on presentation.

Cardiology Board Review: ECG, Hemodynamic and Angiographic Unknowns, First Edition. Edited by George A. Stouffer.
© 2019 John Wiley & Sons Ltd. Published 2019 by John Wiley & Sons Ltd.

complex to the end of the T wave. The QT interval should be measured over 3–5 beats in leads II, V5, and V6 with the longest value being used. The length of QT varies inversely with heart rate and thus the QT interval needs to be "corrected" (QTc). The QT interval also varies with gender and the upper limit of normal for QTc is 0.44–0.45 seconds for males and 0.46–0.47 seconds for females. A very rough rule of thumb is that the QT interval should not be greater than half the RR distance when the rhythm is regular.

The most common method used for correcting QT interval for heart rate is the Bazett formula (QTc = QT/√RR in seconds, with all intervals in seconds). The Bazett formula provides an adequate correction for heart rate ranging anywhere between 60 and 100 beats/min but underestimates and overestimates the QT interval at low and high heart rates, respectively. For heart rates outside the normal range, other correction methods such as Fredericia (QTc = QT/[RR]1/3) or Framingham (QTc = QT + 0.154[1 − RR]) should be utilized. It is important to note that these correction methods are based on population mean correction factor and do not address intra- or interindividual variability.

The QT interval measures the time needed for ventricular depolarization and repolarization but in the presence of a normal QRS duration, long QT intervals occur when there is a prolongation of repolarization. LQTS can be either acquired or genetic. Causes of acquired prolonged QT intervals include severe hypothermia, hypokalemia, severe hypocalcemia, hypothyroidism, antiarrhythmic drug classes IA and III, other medications (e.g. antihistamines, antipsychotics, antibiotics, antidepressants, methadone, etc), severe bradycardia, atrioventricular block, myocardial ischemia, and neurogenic causes (including organophosphorus). Previously unrecognized LQTS is present in 5–20% of patients with drug-induced torsades de pointes.

More than 10 different types of congenital LQTS have been recognized, with LQT1, LQT2, and LQT3 accounting for the vast majority of the cases of congenital LQTS (Table 31.1). Inherited LQTS was first described by Jervell and Lange-Nielsen in 1957 when they reported a family with deafness, LQTS, and recurrent sudden cardiac death. That family was subsequently shown to have a homozygous mutation of KCNQ1 (also known as KVLQT1; a heterozygote mutation in this gene causes LQTS1). A few

Table 31.1 Types of LQTS.

	LQTS1	LQTS2	LQTS3
Gene affected	KCNQ1 (KVLQT1)	KCNH2 (hERG)	SCN5A
Ion channel	Adrenergic-sensitive potassium channel	Potassium channel	Sodium channel
Triggers of syncope and sudden death	Emotional or physical stress (e.g. swimming)	Can occur at stress or rest. Triggering by loud noises is very suggestive of LQTS2	Rest or sleep
Response of QT interval to exercise	Failure to shorten	Normal	Supernormal
T wave	Broad T wave	Low amplitude, bifid T wave	Narrow tall T wave
Frequency	40-55% of LQTS	35-45% of LQTS	8-10% of LQTS
Miscellaneous	Most common form of LQTS	Risk increases during post-partum period	Also associated with bradycardia

years later, Romano et al. and then Ward described long QT, syncope, and sudden cardiac death but with normal hearing. More recent work has shown that LQTS is a disease of cardiac ion channels with clinical manifestations being linked to over 300 mutations in ten different genes. In general, LQTS is caused by a heterozygous mutation and thus inheritance is autosomal dominant with variable penetrance. Mutations in three genes comprise the vast majority of cases and are described below. Homozygous mutations such as described by Jervell and Lang-Nielsen are rare (less than 1% of all LQTS cases) and associated with autosomal recessive inheritance and congenital deafness.

LQTS1 and LQTS2 are caused by mutations in genes that result in a decrease in repolarizing K potassium ion channels. LQTS1 is caused by a mutation in the gene KCNQ1, encoding the ion channel for the slow delayed rectifier potassium current. LQTS2 is caused by a mutation in the gene KCNH2 (also known as hERG), encoding the ion channel for the rapid delayed rectifier potassium current. The mutations can cause the channels to be blocked completely, open after a delay, or close prematurely, thus causing decreased potassium outward current and a longer duration of repolarization. Increased sympathetic stimulation can provoke arrhythmias in LQTS1 and LQTS2 patients. In LQTS1, exercise (especially swimming) and emotional stress can precipitate syncope and sudden cardiac death. Arrhythmic events in LQTS2 can occur at stress or rest; triggering by unexpected loud noises (e.g. alarm clock) is very suggestive of LQTS2. LQTS1 and LQTS2 account for the majority of all LQTS cases.

LQTS3 is caused by mutations of the SCN5A sodium channel gene, leading to delayed closing of the channel, a constant inward sodium current, and prolonged repolarization. LQTS3 accounts for <10% of all LQTS cases and individuals with LQTS3 tend to experience cardiac events while sleeping. LQTS3 can also be associated with bradycardia, and syncopal events can be precipitated by slow heart rates in addition to rapid ventricular arrhythmias.

The three major LQTS genes (KCNQ1, KCNH2, and SCN5A) account for approximately 75% of the disorder. There are 10 minor LQTS-susceptibility genes that collectively account for less than 5% of LQTS cases. In addition, three multisystem disorders associated with QT prolongation have been described, including ankyrin-B syndrome, Anderson-Tawil syndrome (ATS), and Timothy syndrome (TS). LQTS is typically inherited in an autosomal dominant manner except for LQTS associated with sensorineural deafness (known as Jervell and Lange-Nielsen syndrome), which is inherited in an autosomal recessive manner.

In patients with LQTS, the most powerful predictor of risk of arrhythmia is the length of the QTc. In an analysis of more than 600 patients with LQTS 1, 2, or 3, the risk of syncope or sudden cardiac death was >70% if QTc was greater than 498 ms. Other risk factors include age (syncope and sudden death are unusual >40 years old), gender, previous syncope or sudden death, and type of mutation. Genetic testing can be helpful but does not exclude the diagnosis (the individual may have an unrecognized variant).

In this ECG, the QTc is 497 ms. This suggests LQTS and should prompt an evaluation for causes of long QT. Also, a family history of death at an early age should be sought (both in first degree and in distant relatives), with particular attention paid to death from drowning or death due to trauma which could have been caused by syncope (e.g. while driving like in her father). In patients with long QT interval and a clinical diagnosis of syncope or sudden cardiac death, the diagnosis of LQTS can be made. In other patients, a clinical scoring system may be useful. Genetic testing will confirm the diagnosis if the patient has a known mutation, which is the case for approximately 75% of LQTS patients at this time. Echocardiography can be used to eliminate structural cardiac disease. Family screening is indicated if LQTS is diagnosed.

Further Reading

Abrams, D.J. and MacRae, C.A. (2014). Long QT syndrome. *Circulation* 129 (14): 1524–1529.

Nachimuthu, S., Assar, M.D., and Schussler, J.M. (2012). Drug-induced QT interval prolongation: mechanisms and clinical management. *Therapeutic Advances in Drug Safety* 3 (5): 241–253.

Case 32: An Unusual ECG in a Homeless Man Who Is Unconscious

A 25-year-old homeless individual is brought to the Emergency Department after being found unconscious. What clues does the ECG provide in establishing a differential diagnosis (Figure 32.1)?

Hypothermia

This ECG is from a patient suffering from hypothermia, or low core body temperature. The main diagnostic clue is the late positive deflections after the terminal portion of the QRS complex, known as Osborn or J waves (present in the inferior and lateral leads but most prominent in leads V3–V6). Other manifestations of hypothermia on this ECG include prolongation of the PR interval, T wave inversion, increased QT interval duration, and QRS prolongation.

The rhythm is atrial fibrillation. Atrial fibrillation occurs in approximately 50% of patients with hypothermia. Atrial flutter, AV junctional rhythm, ventricular ectopic beats,

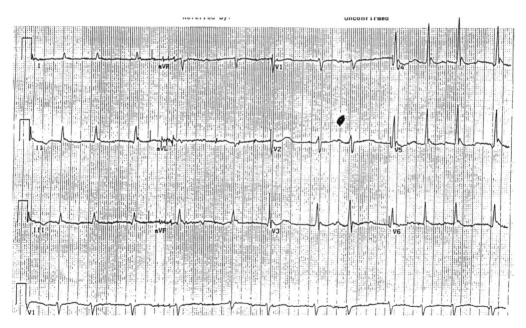

Figure 32.1 ECG on presentation.

Cardiology Board Review: ECG, Hemodynamic and Angiographic Unknowns, First Edition. Edited by George A. Stouffer.
© 2019 John Wiley & Sons Ltd. Published 2019 by John Wiley & Sons Ltd.

and ventricular fibrillation can also occur with hypothermia. Note the artifact indicated by rapid, intermittent oscillations in this ECG. This is often present in hypothermic patients because of shivering.

A distinct inflection in the J point was described by John Osborn in 1953 based on his experiments on cardiac and respiratory function in hypothermic dogs (Osborn 1953). Over the years different names have been applied to this phenomenon including "camel-hump sign," "late delta wave," "hypothermic wave," "J point wave," "K wave," "H wave," and "current of injury" with most current commentators using the term Osborn waves. Osborn thought acidemia induced by hypothermia was the primary cause of the inflection in the J point but subsequent work has shown that a difference in the electrophysiology of the ventricular epicardium and endocardium is the basis for Osborn waves. Specifically, Osborn waves are thought to arise from differences in the transient outward current of the endo- and epicardium during early repolarization.

Osborn waves (Figure 32.2) are commonly seen in the inferior and lateral leads (II, III, aVF, V5, and V6), become more prominent as the body temperature drops, and regress with rewarming. At temperatures below 86°, 80% of patients have Osborn waves. Osborn

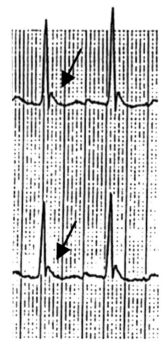

Figure 32.2 Osborn waves.

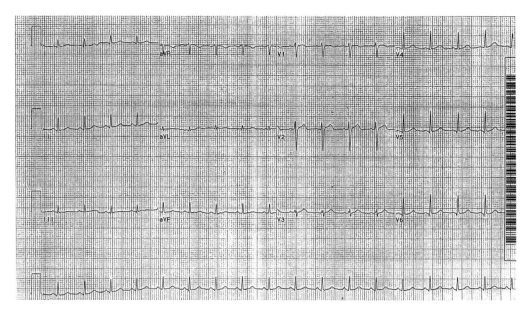

Figure 32.3 ECG after the body temperature had increased showing resolution of the Osborn waves.

waves are traditionally associated with hypothermia but have also been reported in patients with extreme hypercalcemia, acute brain injury, subarachnoid hemorrhage, cardiopulmonary arrest, vasospastic angina, and idiopathic ventricular fibrillation.

ECG changes become more prominent with progressive decreases in temperature. Sinus tachycardia may be the only ECG manifestation of mild hypothermia. If the core body temperature continues to drop, sinus bradycardia supervenes and is associated with progressive prolongation of the PR interval, QRS complex, and QT interval. Further decreases in temperature are often associated with premature atrial contractions and/or atrial fibrillation. With temperature <86°F, a progressive widening of the QRS complex increases the risk of ventricular fibrillation. When the temperature drops to 60°F, asystole supervenes.

The Osborn waves in this patient resolved and sinus rhythm returned as his body temperature increased (Figure 32.3).

Further Reading

Chhabra, L., Devadoss, R., Liti, B. et al. (2013). Electrocardiographic changes in hypothermia: a review. *Therapeutic Hypothermia and Temperature Management* 3 (2): 54–62.

Osborn, J.J. (1953). Experimental Hypothermia: Respiratory and Blood pH Changes in Relation to Cardiac Function. *American Journal of Physiology* 175: 389–398.

Case 33: An 18-Year-Old Student with Fever, Chest Pain, and ST Elevation

You are asked to see an 18-year-old male with no past medical history who presented to the Emergency Department with sudden onset of chest pain. He states that he woke from sleep at 4:30a.m. the day of a presentation with sharp substernal chest pain with no clear exacerbating or alleviating factors. He took ibuprofen without relief, so he decided to seek medical attention. He has no prior cardiac history but reports that for two days prior to his presentation he was ill with an upper respiratory tract infection consisting of fever (temperature of 101°F), chills, cough, congestion, and myalgias.

On exam in the emergency department he is afebrile, heart rate is 57 beats per minute, blood pressure is 130/82 mmHg, and he has a normal respiratory rate and oxygen saturation. He appears uncomfortable. His breath sounds are equal bilaterally and without wheezes, rales, or rhonchi. Cardiac exam reveals regular rate and rhythm, and no rub is appreciated. He has 2+ distal pulses in all extremities and no peripheral edema.

His ECG on presentation is shown below (Figure 33.1). What is the diagnosis?

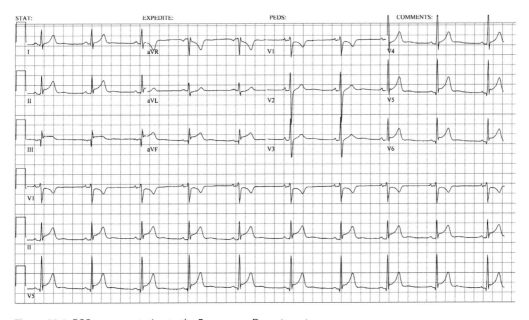

Figure 33.1 ECG on presentation to the Emergency Department.

Cardiology Board Review: ECG, Hemodynamic and Angiographic Unknowns, First Edition. Edited by George A. Stouffer.
© 2019 John Wiley & Sons Ltd. Published 2019 by John Wiley & Sons Ltd.

Additional Evaluation

The ECG showed sinus bradycardia with diffuse ST elevation in inferior and lateral leads. Initial lab work was remarkable for troponin 30.9 ng/ml, creatinine kinase of 735 U/L, CK-MB of 62.2 U/L, white blood cell count of 12.6 × 10⁹ cells/L, and C-reactive protein of 2.3 mg/L. Bedside ultrasound was completed in the Emergency Department which showed normal left ventricular and right ventricular function, no significant valvular pathology, and no pericardial effusion. He was admitted with the presumptive diagnosis of myopericarditis and treated with anti-inflammatory medications.

His hospital course was unremarkable, and he improved quickly with medical therapy. Viral panel returned positive for rhinovirus/enterovirus. His cardiac troponin peaked at 73.9 ng/ml. His ECG showed persistence of ST elevation for 24 hours with eventual development of T wave inversions diffusely (Figure 33.2). Repeat echocardiogram showed no changes. He was discharged on oral ibuprofen with scheduled outpatient follow-up.

Myopericarditis

Myopericarditis involves inflammation of both the myocardium and pericardium. In general, this is primarily a pericardial inflammatory syndrome with relatively mild myocardial involvement (Imazio and Cooper 2013), but it should be noted that there is a wide spectrum of disease and varying amounts of myocardial injury are observed. In order to diagnose myopericarditis, a diagnosis of pericarditis must be fulfilled based on two or more of the following: chest pain, friction rub on cardiac auscultation, widespread ST elevation or PR depression on ECG, and new or worsening pericardial effusion (Imazio et al. 2013). Myocardial involvement is suspected based on elevated cardiac markers of injury (troponin, CK-MB fraction), or a new focal wall motion abnormality or diffusely depressed left ventricular (LV) function by echocardiogram or cardiac MRI (magnetic resonance imaging) (Imazio et al. 2013).

The etiology of myopericarditis falls into one of three categories: idiopathic, infectious, or immune related (Imazio and Cooper 2013). In developed countries such as the US, idiopathic causes are thought to typically be related to viral infections and are among the most common causes of myopericarditis, whereas in developing countries tuberculosis is a major cause. (Imazio et al. 2015) The most common viruses suspected of causing myopericarditis are enteroviruses (coxsackie viruses, echoviruses), herpes viruses (Epstein–Barr virus, cytomegalovirus, human herpes virus 6), and adenoviruses. There is also a spectrum of noninfectious causes which are primarily metabolic and traumatic in nature, but autoimmune, neoplastic, and drug-related conditions can also cause a similar presentation (Imazio et al. 2015).

The clinical presentation of myopericarditis reflects the degree of myopericardial involvement. Many patients have mild

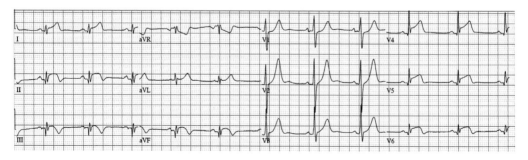

Figure 33.2 ECG obtained 24 hours after presentation.

symptoms, and often cardiac symptoms are preceded or concomitant with a respiratory infection or gastroenteritis (Imazio and Cooper 2013). Commonly, patients complain of positional or pleuritic chest pain which is often difficult to distinguish from ischemic pain. Patients frequently also complain of fever, fatigue, decreased exercise capacity, and palpitations.

The electrocardiogram can be particularly useful in diagnosing myopericarditis. Frequently, patients with myopericarditis have widespread upward concave ST segment elevation that mimics ST elevation myocardial infarction (STEMI) (Lange and Hillis 2004). Because STEMI needs to be treated emergently with revascularization, it is important to distinguish these two entities. PR depression, most frequently noted in lead II, can be a useful tool that is frequently observed in myopericarditis but absent in myocardial ischemia (Lange and Hillis 2004; Porela et al. 2012). Over time, the ST segment normalizes and is replaced by T wave inversions, and finally returns to normal over the course of days to weeks (Chan et al. 1999).

There are four stages of ECG changes associated with the evolution of acute (myo) pericarditis (Table 33.1). Stage 1 changes accompany the onset of chest pain and include the "classic" ECG changes associated with acute pericarditis: diffuse concave ST elevation with PR depression. The ST segment elevation (usually of 1–2 mm) is generally widespread and concave upward. PR depression is generally most evident in lead II, although it can be seen in other leads. Stage 2

occurs several days later and is represented by the return of ST segments to baseline and T wave flattening. In Stage 3, T wave inversion is seen in most leads, especially those in which ST elevation was present in Stage 1. Stage 4 represents the return of upright T waves. The approximate time frame for passage through all four stages of ECG changes in most cases of acute pericarditis is two weeks.

ECG abnormalities are present in approximately 90% of patients with acute pericarditis but only approximately 50% of patients will manifest all four stages. Other ECG presentations include isolated PR depression, absence of one or more stages, or persistence of T wave inversion. Sinus tachycardia may be present and atrial arrhythmias are seen in 5–10% of cases. One last important point: There are no ECG findings that are diagnostic of pericarditis. The ECG must be interpreted in light of the clinical scenario.

Cardiac troponin can be utilized in combination with imaging modalities to determine the extent of myocardial involvement in a patient presenting with symptoms consistent with pericarditis. Troponin elevation indicates myocardial inflammation and is often elevated in the absence of CK-MB; typically serum cardiac troponin returns to normal in less than two weeks. (Imazio and Cooper 2013) Echocardiography is used to evaluate LV function and to assess for the presence of a pericardial effusion, which is part of the diagnostic criteria for pericarditis (Lange and Hillis 2004; Imazio and Cooper 2013). LV function is generally described as mild, global, or segmental decrease in cases of myocardial involvement, though severe cases are also observed (Imazio and Cooper 2013).

Cardiac magnetic resonance imaging (CMR) has proven to have high diagnostic accuracy for the presence of myocardial inflammation. CMR assessment of right and left ventricular function is very reproducible and thus allows for identifying and quantifying even mild functional abnormalities. Additionally, it can allow for detection of edema which is an important marker for inflammatory cell injury. T2 weighted

Table 33.1 Stages of ECG changes in acute myopericarditis.

Stage	ECG Findings
1	ST elevation, PR depression.
2	ST segments return to baseline. There may be diffuse T wave flattening.
3	T wave inversion.
4	Normalization of ECG.

imaging is able to detect tissue edema with high sensitivity, though this does not necessarily distinguish inflammation from ischemia. Myocardial early gadolinium enhancement is especially useful in clinically suspected acute and chronic myocarditis; regional vasodilation is a key feature of inflammation, and increased blood volume in the inflamed area leads to increased uptake of contrast during the early vascular phase. Gadolinium distributes quickly into the interstitial space after administration, so this phase lasts for the first few minutes after the contrast bolus. T1-weighted MR during this time can assess myocardial hyperemia (Friedrich et al. 2009). Late gadolinium enhancement (LGE) indicates areas of myocardial necrosis and fibrosis and indicates areas of permanently damaged tissue in the setting of myocarditis; as a general rule, the subendocardium typically is not involved in an isolated fashion in myopericarditis which can be used to distinguish it from ischemia-mediated injury (Friedrich et al. 2009).

Definitive diagnosis is made on the basis of myocardial biopsy although this is rarely used. Typically, biopsy is only performed in patients with symptomatic LV dysfunction refractory to conventional therapy, or in patients with sustained arrhythmias. Biopsy should be pursued in any patient with a possible diagnosis of giant cell myocarditis, as these patients often require advanced therapies for survival (Imazio and Cooper 2013)

Treatment of idiopathic myopericarditis involves use of empiric anti-inflammatory therapies. Aspirin or NSAIDS (nonsteroidal anti-inflammatory drugs) are considered first-line treatment, while corticosteroids can also be used. Colchicine has not been proven to be efficacious in the setting of myopericarditis despite its benefit in pericarditis. In the case of known bacterial, neoplastic, or rheumatologic conditions causing myopericarditis, treatment should be aimed at these specific conditions. Additionally, rest and avoidance of physical activity beyond normal sedentary activity is recommended during the acute and healing phases of myopericarditis (Imazio and Cooper 2013; Imazio et al. 2013).

References

Chan, T.C., Brady, W.J., and Pollack, M. (1999). Electrocardiographic manifestations: acute myopericarditis. *The Journal of Emergency Medicine* 17 (5): 865–872.

Friedrich, M.G., Sechtem, U., Schulz-Menger, J. et al. (2009). Cardiovascular magnetic resonance in myocarditis: a JACC white paper. *Journal of the American College of Cardiology* 53 (17): 1475–1487.

Imazio, M., Brucato, A., Barbieri, A. et al. (2013). Good prognosis for pericarditis with and without myocardial involvement: results from a multicenter, prospective cohort study. *Circulation* 128 (1): 42–49.

Imazio, M. and Cooper, L.T. (2013). Management of myopericarditis. *Expert Review of Cardiovascular Therapy* 11 (2): 193–201.

Imazio, M., Gaita, F., and LeWinter, M. (2015). Evaluation and treatment of pericarditis: a systematic review. *JAMA* 314 (14): 1498–1506.

Lange, R.A. and Hillis, L.D. (2004). Clinical practice. Acute pericarditis. *The New England Journal of Medicine* 351 (21): 2195–2202.

Porela, P., Kytö, V., Nikus, K. et al. (2012). PR depression is useful in the differential diagnosis of myopericarditis and ST elevation myocardial infarction. *Annals of Noninvasive Electrocardiology* 17 (2): 141–145.

Case 34: Recurrent Endocarditis in a 26-Year-Old Woman

A 26-year-old female with a past medical history of aortic valve endocarditis resulting in placement of a bioprosthetic valve three years ago, acute kidney injury, anxiety, hypertension, chronic back pain, and hepatitis C presented with a three-day history of malaise, generalized weakness, intermittent sweats, chills, subjective fever, and persistent nausea associated with bilious emesis. On cardiac auscultation, there was a normal S1, S2, a regular rate and rhythm, and a III/IV diastolic murmur that was heard best at the right second intercostal space. No obvious conjunctival hemorrhages were appreciated but there were two erythematous areas in her right lower lid. Petechial-like lesions were present on her left thigh that appeared to be resolving, and no tender nodules were present on her hands or feet. Transthoracic echocardiography showed normal left ventricular ejection fraction (55–60%), severe aortic regurgitation, mild mitral and tricuspid regurgitation, mild biatrial enlargement, and a freely mobile echo density attached to the aortic valve that was seen on the aortic side and was suspicious for a vegetation.

What are the most likely bacteria causing infective endocarditis in this patient?

Endocarditis

The microbiology of prosthetic valve endocarditis depends upon the time since implantation. Within two months of surgery, *Staphylococcus aureus*, coagulase-negative staphylococci, gram-negative bacilli, and fungal infection are the most common agents. Infective Endocarditis (IE) cases presenting more than 12 months after valve surgery have the same microbiology spectrum as native valve endocarditis with the most frequently encountered pathogens being streptococci (especially viridans), *S. aureus*, coagulase-negative staphylococci, and enterococci. Cases that present between 2 and 12 months after surgery are a blend of nosocomial and community-acquired infections. Culture-negative cases can occur at any time point after valve surgery.

Background

IE is an infection of the endocardial surface of the heart that can present as either acute or subacute disease. Acute IE presents with a sepsis-like picture including high fever, rigors, and elevated white blood cell count. In contrast, subacute infective endocarditis presents with nonspecific symptoms such as fatigue, dyspnea, or weight loss over several weeks to months. Fever may or may not be present. Physical examination findings may include a new heart murmur due to valve regurgitation, Janeway lesions (non-tender, small erythematous or haemorrhagic macular or nodular lesions on the palms of the hands or soles of the feet), Osler nodes (painful, red, raised lesions found on the hands and feet) or other evidence of system embolization.

Cardiology Board Review: ECG, Hemodynamic and Angiographic Unknowns, First Edition. Edited by George A. Stouffer.
© 2019 John Wiley & Sons Ltd. Published 2019 by John Wiley & Sons Ltd.

Risk factors for developing IE include age > 60 years old, male gender, prior IE, existence of a prosthetic valve or cardiac device, history of valvular or congenital heart disease, chronic hemodialysis, intravenous drug use, indwelling intravenous lines, skin infection, immunosuppression, and recent dental or surgical procedure(Wallace et al. 2002; Hasbun et al. 2003; Chu et al. 2004; Hill et al. 2007; Wang et al. 2007). The six-month mortality rate among IE patients can be as high as 27%.

Clinical Presentation

Any organ system can be involved in patients with IE, and thus the clinical presentation can be highly variable depending on the microorganism and risk factors involved. The classic signs and symptoms of IE include fever, bacteremia or fungemia, valvular incompetence, peripheral emboli, and immune-mediated vasculitis as is seen in subacute IE. However, in cases of acute IE that evolve too quickly for immunologic phenomena to develop, patients may present only with fever or severe manifestations, such as those related to valve incompetency.

It is sometimes possible to make the diagnosis of IE clinically with a careful physical examination. Cases involving patients presenting with a new onset murmur or worsening murmur with signs of infection or bacteremia are highly suggestive of IE (Selton-Suty et al. 2012; Cahill and Prendergast 2016). Janeway lesions, which are painless, erythematous macules found on the palms and soles, and Osler nodes, which are painful lesions found on the fingers and toes, are rare, yet also highly indicative of IE when present. Retinal hemorrhages known as Roth's spots, conjunctival hemorrhages, signs of CHF, splenomegaly, petechiae, splinter hemorrhages, and septic emboli are additional physical examination findings suggestive of IE. Clinical presentation can be further supported by several nonspecific, yet suggestive laboratory studies. Laboratory findings in IE include anemia, thrombocytopenia, leukocytosis, active urinary sediment, elevated sedimentation rate, hypergammaglobulinemia, positive rheumatoid factor, antinuclear antibodies, hypocomplementemia, and false-positive Venereal Disease Research Laboratory and Lyme disease serology (Weickert et al. 2019).

Diagnosis and Management

The diagnosis of IE should be considered in patients presenting with fever, either with or without bacteremia, relevant cardiac risk factors, or noncardiac risk factors. Once IE is suspected, the diagnosis is confirmed with clinical manifestations, blood cultures (or other microbiologic findings), and transthoracic echocardiography (Hill et al. 2007). Other evaluative methods for patients include electrocardiography, chest radiography, other radiographic imaging depending on clinical manifestations, and dental evaluation.

The modified Duke criteria is used to diagnose IE. Definitive IE is established with: (i) two major criteria; (ii) one major criterion and three minor criteria; or (iii) five minor criteria. IE may also be diagnosed by either the presence of vegetations or intracardiac abscess demonstrating active endocarditis on histology or by finding select microorganisms by culture or histology of a vegetation or intracardiac abscess (Durack et al. 1994; Prendergast 2004).

Major criteria include: (i) at least two separate positive blood cultures for agents associated with IE; and (ii) echocardiographic evidence for IE including an oscillating intracardiac mass on a valve or supporting structures, abscess, new partial dehiscence of prosthetic valve, or new valvular regurgitation (worsening or changing of preexisting murmur not sufficient). Minor criteria include: (i) predisposition, predisposing heart condition, or injection drug use; (ii) temperature of more than 38 °C; (iii) evidence of system embolization of emboli such as septic pulmonary infarcts, mycotic aneurysm, intracranial hemorrhage, conjunctival hemorrhages, and Janeway lesions; (iv) immunologic phenomena such as glomerulonephritis, Osler nodes, Roth spots, and rheumatoid factor; and (v) positive blood culture but does not meet a major criterion as noted above or serological evidence of active infection with organism consistent with infective endocarditis.

Prior to the administration of antibiotics, three sets of blood cultures should be obtained from three different venipuncture sites. If the patient is stable, antibiotics should be administered after the results of blood cultures and diagnostic tests are determined to decrease the chance of false-negative results. However, if the patient is unstable, antibiotics should be administered

while awaiting results (Weickert et al. 2019). In general, empiric therapy should cover methicillin-susceptible and methicillin-resistant staphylococci, streptococci, and enterococci. Vancomycin is commonly used as empiric therapy (Wilson et al. 1984; Stevens and Edmond 2005; Dahl et al. 2013). After initial empiric therapy, antimicrobial agents should be selected based on the causative microbe.

After a diagnosis is made, echocardiography is also useful for identifying patients at high risk for complications and assessing the need for surgery. Vegetations larger than 10 mm, heart failure unresponsive to therapy, new heart block, and vegetations that increase in size while on therapy are findings that indicate increased risk of complications and/or the need for surgery. Finally, follow-up blood cultures should always be performed to assure eradication of bacteremia after therapy (Weickert et al. 2019).

References

Cahill, T.J. and Prendergast, B.D. (2016). Infective endocarditis. *Lancet* 387: 882.

Chu, V.H., Cabell, C.H., Benjamin, D.K. Jr. et al. (2004). Early predictors of in-hospital death in infective endocarditis. *Circulation* 109: 1745.

Dahl, A., Rasmussen, R.V., Bundgaard, H. et al. (2013). Enterococcus faecalis infective endocarditis: a pilot study of the relationship between duration of gentamicin treatment and outcome. *Circulation* 127: 1810.

Durack, D.T., Lukes, A.S., and Bright, D.K. (1994). New criteria for diagnosis of infective endocarditis: utilization of specific echocardiographic findings. Duke Endocarditis Service. *The American Journal of Medicine* 96: 200.

Hasbun, R., Vikram, H.R., Barakat, L.A. et al. (2003). Complicated left-sided native valve endocarditis in adults: risk classification for mortality. *JAMA* 289: 1933.

Hill, E.E., Herijgers, P., Claus, P. et al. (2007). Infective endocarditis: changing epidemiology and predictors of 6-month mortality: a prospective cohort study. *European Heart Journal* 28: 196.

Prendergast, B.D. (2004). Diagnostic criteria and problems in infective endocarditis. *Heart* 90: 611.

Selton-Suty, C., Célard, M., Le Moing, V. et al. (2012). Preeminence of Staphylococcus aureus in infective endocarditis: a 1-year population-based survey. *Clinical Infectious Diseases* 54: 1230.

Stevens, M.P. and Edmond, M.B. (2005). Endocarditis due to vancomycin-resistant enterococci: case report and review of the literature. *Clinical Infectious Diseases* 41: 1134.

Weickert, T.T., Patterson, K.B. and Patterson C. Infective Endocarditis in Netters Cardiology, ed. Stouffer, G.A., Runge, M.S., Patterson, C., Rossi, J.S., et al. (2019). Elsevier.

Wallace, S.M., Walton, B.I., Kharbanda, R.K. et al. (2002). Mortality from infective endocarditis: clinical predictors of outcome. *Heart* 88: 53.

Wang, A., Athan, E., Pappas, P.A. et al. (2007). Contemporary clinical profile and outcome of prosthetic valve endocarditis. *JAMA* 297: 1354.

Wilson, W.R., Wilkowske, C.J., Wright, A.J. et al. (1984). Treatment of streptomycin-susceptible and streptomycin-resistant enterococcal endocarditis. *Annals of Internal Medicine* 100: 816.

Case 35: A 23-Year-Old Man with a Loud Systolic Murmur

A 23-year-old male with Trisomy 21 and history of a childhood cardiac surgery is referred to you for evaluation of a heart murmur. He is accompanied by his mother who helps provide the history. The patient recently moved with his family from a different health system and established care with a new primary care provider who noticed the presence of a systolic murmur. No surgical procedure notes are available but his mother reports, "they closed a hole in his heart."

Physical examination reveals a pleasant, short, obese male in no acute distress. He is noted to have a short neck with a prominent tongue. Examination of his extremities demonstrates broad, short hands with a long, single midline crease on his palms. On careful auscultation, aortic and pulmonic components of the second heart sound remain split during both inspiration and expiration. A III/VI holosystolic murmur is observed at the mid-axilla. Laboratory panel shows normal complete blood count, metabolic panel, and thyroid function. What clues can you derive from the electrocardiogram (Figure 35.1)?

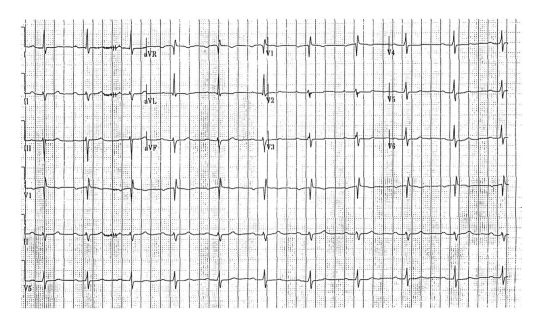

Figure 35.1 ECG in a 23-year-old male with a systolic murmur.

Cardiology Board Review: ECG, Hemodynamic and Angiographic Unknowns, First Edition. Edited by George A. Stouffer.
© 2019 John Wiley & Sons Ltd. Published 2019 by John Wiley & Sons Ltd.

Ostium Primum Atrial Septal Defect

This patient's constellation of symptoms, physical exam findings, and clinical tests are representative of a previously repaired ostium primum atrial septal defect (ASD) and repaired ventricular septal defect. Primum septal defects are frequently recognized in early childhood, particularly when present alongside other congenital heart abnormalities. Primum ASDs can specifically occur concurrently with ventricular septal defects due to common pathophysiology, with both abnormalities involving the endocardial cushions. In this case, thickening of the high ventricular septum and interatrial septum suggest his childhood cardiac surgery involved the closing of a relatively large shunt. Additionally, his moderate mitral regurgitation may be representative of a cleft anterior mitral leaflet (A2 segment most commonly), another condition sometimes observed with primum ASDs. Finally, patients with Trisomy 21 (Down syndrome) have an increased incidence of atrioventricular septal defects.

ECG findings associated with an ostium primum ASD are similar to those seen with an ostium secundum ASD with the major exception being left axis deviation. An rSr′ or rsR′ pattern in lead V1 is common. In addition, there maybe first-degree AV block. Since most ostium primum ASDs are relatively large (causing significant left-to-right shunts) and associated with mitral regurgitation because of abnormalities in the mitral valve, right ventricular hypertrophy and/or right atrial abnormalities are common. The incidence of atrial arrhythmias increases with age and becomes common after 30 years.

A transthoracic echocardiogram showed evidence of thickening in the high interventricular septum consistent with previous surgical ventricular septal defect closure. There is also evidence of previous atrial septal defect closure. Colorflow Doppler imaging reveals moderate mitral regurgitation.

Clinical Presentation

Atrial septal defect is the most common congenital cardiac abnormality in adults in the United States (Linde et al. 2011). There are four types of atrial septal defects – ostium primum, ostium secundum, sinus venosus, and coronary sinus defects. After secundum ASDs (75% of cases), primum ASDs are the next most common comprising 15–20% of cases (Stout et al. 2018). Since many primum septal defects are recognized in childhood, most patients who present as adults were those in whom a small ASD was not corrected or a larger defect was previously surgically corrected. In a small ASD (<5 mm), this shunting may be clinically insignificant (Craig and Selzer 1968). However, moderate-to-large ASDs can result in more substantial left-to-right shunting, resulting in right ventricular volume overload, right ventricular dilation, and right atrial enlargement. Patients may then go on to develop atrial arrhythmias secondary to atrial stretch and fibrosis. They may also complain of shortness of breath as well as other signs of right heart failure – fluid retention, hepatosplenomegaly, and elevated jugular venous distension. If this condition remains uncorrected, pulmonary artery pressures can dramatically rise, leading to suprasystemic levels and finally result in right-to-left shunting (Eisenmenger's syndrome).

Pathophysiology

During normal embryologic development, the atrial septum is formed by the caudal growth of the septum primum from the superior aspect of the atrium until it reaches the endocardial cushions. A primum septal defect is present in circumstances where the septum primum fails to reach and fuse with the endocardial cushions. The clinical presentation and subsequent clinical ramifications of primum ASD depend largely on the size and extent of shunting.

Diagnosis

Most primum ASDs are recognized by transthoracic echocardiography and are associated with other cardiac congenital abnormalities included ventricular septal defect and cleft mitral leaflet. As such, most patients with a history of primum ASD have had surgical closure by the time they encounter a cardiologist as an adult.

On physical examination, a widely, fixed split second heart sound may be observed. During normal physiology, inspiration leads to increased right-sided cardiac filling with resulting delayed closure of the pulmonic valve and a split second heart sound. This effect disappears with expiration as the aortic and pulmonic valves close at relatively the same time. In the presence of a left-to-right shunt with a primum ASD, S2 remains split as during expiration, blood flow from the left heart results in increased right ventricular filling and once again delays the closure of the pulmonic valve. Additionally, a holosystolic, blowing murmur may be auscultated in the axilla due mitral regurgitation in those patients with an associated cleft anterior leaflet mitral leaflet.

Comprehensive echocardiography is invaluable in the diagnosis of primum ASDs. In addition to visualization of the defect, transthoracic echocardiography can be helpful in quantifying pulmonary artery pressures and estimating shunt magnitude. In certain circumstances, it may be difficult to differentiate a primum ASD from a particularly caudal secundum ASD. However, certain associated echocardiographic findings can help point to the correct anatomical diagnosis. In normal hearts, the tricuspid valve is usually apically displaced approximately 10–15 mm from corresponding atrioventricular groove of the mitral valve. This apical displacement is generally preserved in those patients with a secundum ASD. Conversely, the tricuspid and mitral valves are usually located at the same level in patients with primum ASD.

Transesophageal echocardiography is a useful adjunct to measure septal defect margins in multiple dimensions and allow for planning of surgical ASD closure. Magnetic resonance imaging is not required for the evaluation of all ASDs but can be used to further quantify shunt severity.

Management

Appropriate and timely recognition of a primum ASD is crucial. The most recent ACC/AHA (American College of Cardiology/American Heart Association) guidelines for the diagnosis of atrial septal defects contain a class 1 indication to employ an imaging technique to diagnose ASD and/or refer to a center with the capability to do so in those patients with unexplained right ventricular volume overload (Stout et al. 2018).

Unlike secundum ASDs, percutaneous closure of primum ASDs should be avoided. In those patients with right atrial or right ventricular enlargement, surgical correction of primum ASDs is recommended (class 1) (Stout 2018). ASD closure is reasonable in patients who present with paradoxical embolism or with orthodeoxia-playtpnea (class 2a) (Stout 2018). ASD closure is contraindicated in patients with severe, irreversible pulmonary arterial hypertension and no evidence of left-to-right shunt (class 3) (Stout 2018). During follow-up visits, the patient should be evaluated for development of new arrhythmias and pulmonary pressures, and right ventricular function and residual shunting should be assessed. Presence of a pericardial effusion and/or cardiac tamponade should be considered particularly in the days to weeks after surgical closure. Additionally, in those patients who develop atrial fibrillation as a consequence of an ASD, cardioversion after appropriate anticoagulation is recommended to restore sinus rhythm; rate control and anticoagulation is recommended if rhythm control cannot be achieved (class 1) (Stout 2018).

References

Craig, R.J. and Selzer, A. (1968). Natural history and prognosis of atrial septal defect. *Circulation* 37: 805–815.

Stout, K.K., Daniels, C.J., Aboulhosn, J.A. et al. (2018). 2018 AHA/ACC guideline for the management of adults with congenital heart disease: a report of the American College of Cardiology/American Heart Association Task Force on Clinical Practice Guidelines. *Journal of the American College of Cardiology* 73: 1494–1563. https://doi.org/10.1016/j.jacc.2018.08.1028.

Van der Linde, D., Konings, E.E., Slager, M.A. et al. (2011). Birth prevalence of congenital heart disease worldwide: a systematic review and meta-analysis. *Journal of the American College of Cardiology* 58: 2241–2247.

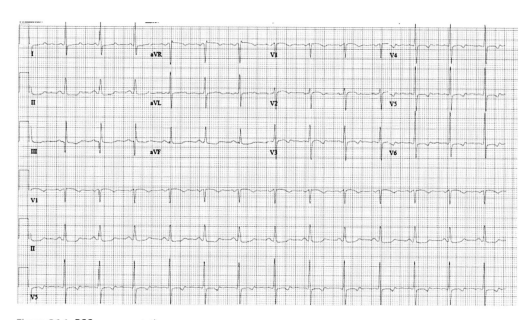

Case 36: A 66-Year-Old Woman with Dyspnea for Two Weeks Which Has Now Abruptly Worsened

A 66-year-old female with a history of treated hypertension presents to the Emergency Department via Emergency Medical System transport. She reports progressive dyspnea over the past few weeks, with sudden worsening tonight while walking to the bathroom. What clues does the ECG provide in establishing a differential diagnosis (Figure 36.1)?

Pulmonary Embolus

Electrocardiographic abnormalities, including unexplained tachycardia, are common in acute pulmonary embolus (PE) but nonspecific.

The ECG is abnormal in over 70% of patients with PE, with sinus tachycardia being the most common abnormality. Other ECG findings generally relate to the effect of the PE on right ventricular (RV) and right atrial pressure and function and may include right bundle branch block (RBBB), large R wave in lead V1, right axis deviation, T wave inversion in leads V1 to V4, P pulmonale, and/or atrial arrhythmias. The combination of an S wave in lead I and a Q wave and inverted T wave in lead III gives the $S_IQ_{III}T_{III}$ pattern suggestive of right ventricular strain. This ECG pattern has been reported to occur in 12% of patients with massive PE.

Figure 36.1 ECG on presentation.

Cardiology Board Review: ECG, Hemodynamic and Angiographic Unknowns, First Edition. Edited by George A. Stouffer.
© 2019 John Wiley & Sons Ltd. Published 2019 by John Wiley & Sons Ltd.

Numerous other ECG findings have also been reported in PE.

All of these findings are nonspecific and the ECG is neither sensitive nor specific for the diagnosis of pulmonary embolus. Roger et al. studied the diagnostic value of 30 different ECG changes in 246 patients with suspected PE. They found that tachycardia and incomplete RBBB were the only ECG findings that were significantly more common in patients with proven PE. The positive predictive value of tachycardia and incomplete RBBB were 38 and 100% respectively. Acute changes of RV overload can also be seen in other conditions such as pneumonia or acute exacerbation of chronic obstructive pulmonary disease.

In contrast to limited usefulness in diagnosing PE, some studies have shown prognostic information can be derived from the ECG in patients with known PE. The presence of low voltage, atrial fibrillation, and/or premature ventricular extrasystoles have been associated with increased 30-day mortality. A 21-point ECG scoring system has been developed that predicts RV dysfunction in patients with acute PE, although the ability to predict in-hospital outcomes is limited. ECG abnormalities have been observed to return to normal after treatment for PE and resolution of anterior T wave changes has been linked to an improved prognosis.

Further Reading

Daniel, K.R., Courtney, D.M., and Kline, J.A. (2001). Assessment of cardiac stress from massive pulmonary embolism with 12-lead ECG. *Chest* 120: 474–481.

Ferrari, E., Imbert, A., Chevalier, T. et al. (1997). The ECG in pulmonary embolism: predictive value of negative T waves in precordial leads: 80 case reports. *Chest* 111: 537–543.

Iles, S., Le Heron, C.J., Davies, G. et al. (2004). ECG score predicts those with the greatest percentage of perfusion defects due to acute pulmonary thromboembolic disease. *Chest* 125: 1651–1656.

Rodger, M., Makropoulos, D., Turek, M. et al. (2000). Diagnostic value of the electrocardiogram in suspected pulmonary embolism. *The American Journal of Cardiology* 86: 807–809.

Stein, P.D., Terrin, M.L., Hales, C.A. et al. (1991). Clinical, laboratory, roentgenographic, and electrocardiographic findings in patients with acute pulmonary embolism and no pre-existing cardiac or pulmonary disease. *Chest* 100: 598–603.

Toosi, M.S., Merlino, J.D., and Leeper, K.V. (2007). Electrocardiographic score and short-term outcomes of acute pulmonary embolism. *The American Journal of Cardiology* 100: 1172–1176.

Case 37: An Unusual Ventriculogram

The following imaging is obtained during an injection of contrast into the left ventricle on a 46-year-old female undergoing evaluation for dyspnea on exertion (Figure 37.1). What is the diagnosis?

Ventricular Septal Defect

Contrast can be seen opacifying the right ventricle during the injection, indicating a connection between the two ventricles (Figure 37.2).

Ventricular septal defects (VSD) are a common congenital heart defect and account for

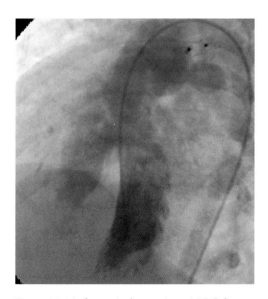

Figure 37.1 Left ventriculogram in an LAO (left anterior oblique) projection.

approximately 10% of congenital heart disease diagnosed in adults. They vary greatly in location, clinical presentation, associated lesions, and natural history. They can be associated with other congenital anomalies including atrial septal defect, patent ductus arteriosus, right aortic arch, and pulmonary stenosis. Multiple VSDs occur but usually in association with complex congenital heart disease. In young adults, concomitant aortic insufficiency may be present in patients with VSDs and indicates a worse prognosis.

There are various nomenclatures used to label the location of a VSD. In brief, VSDs can be classified based on anatomic location as either membranous, muscular, inlet, or infundibular. True membranous septal defects are surrounded by fibrous tissue. Defects that involve the membranous septum and extend into the muscular portion of the septum are called perimembranous. The trabecular septum is the largest part of the interventricular septum. Muscular VSDs within the trabecular septum can undergo spontaneous closure as a result of muscular occlusion. The inlet portion of the septum begins at the level of the atrioventricular (AV) valves and defects in the inlet septum can include abnormalities of the tricuspid and mitral valves (e.g. AV canal defects). The infundibular septum separates the right and left ventricular outflow tracts. The majority of VSDs in adults are perimembranous.

This patient had a small VSD with predominant left-to-right shunting (Qp/Qs = 1.2). No treatment was needed at this point in time.

Cardiology Board Review: ECG, Hemodynamic and Angiographic Unknowns, First Edition. Edited by George A. Stouffer.
© 2019 John Wiley & Sons Ltd. Published 2019 by John Wiley & Sons Ltd.

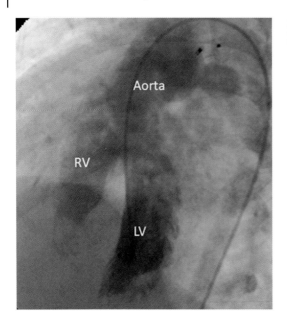

Figure 37.2 Left ventriculogram in an LAO projection (RV = right ventricle; LV = left ventricle).

Further Reading

Brickner, M.E., Hillis, L.D. and Lange, R.A., (2000). Congenital heart disease in adults. *New England Journal of Medicine*, 342(5): 334–342.

Fitzsimmons, S. and Salmon, A. (2018). Congenital heart disease in adults. *Medicine*. 46: 698–702.

Pandya, B., Cullen, S., and Walker, F. (2016). Congenital heart disease in adults. *BMJ* 354: i3905.

Penny, D. J., and Vick III, G. W. (2011). Ventricular septal defect. *The Lancet*. 377(9771): 1103–1112.

Stout, K.K., Daniels, C.J., Aboulhosn, J.A. et al. (2018 Aug 10). 2018 AHA/ACC guideline for the management of adults with congenital heart disease: a report of the American College of Cardiology/ American Heart Association Task Force on Clinical Practice Guidelines. *Journal of the American College of Cardiology* 73: 1494– 1563. https://doi.org/10.1016/j. jacc.2018.08.1028.

Case 38: A 68-Year-Old Male with Generalized Weakness and Dyspnea

You are referred a 68-year-old male with a past medical history of multiple myeloma, hypertension, diabetes mellitus, chronic kidney disease, and diastolic dysfunction who reports generalized weakness and dyspnea that had been ongoing for several months. He had also experienced intermittent palpitations that were not necessarily brought on by physical activity.

On physical examination, his blood pressure is 105/70 mmHg, heart rate is 82 bpm, and oxygen saturation is 93% on room air. He has jugular venous dissension but no carotid artery bruits. His lungs have rales at the bases. Cardiovascular examination shows normal S1 and S2 without any murmurs. He has significant bilateral peripheral edema halfway up his shin.

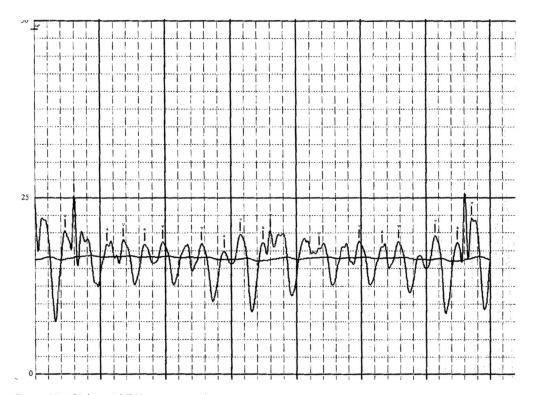

Figure 38.1 Right atrial (RA) pressure tracing.

Cardiology Board Review: ECG, Hemodynamic and Angiographic Unknowns, First Edition. Edited by George A. Stouffer.
© 2019 John Wiley & Sons Ltd. Published 2019 by John Wiley & Sons Ltd.

An echocardiogram showed left ventricular hypertrophy, normal left ventricular ejection fraction, and a small pericardial effusion. Coronary angiography was normal. Mildly decreased cardiac output was identified with a cardiac output of 3.17l per minute by Assumed Fick calculation. Right atrial (RA) pressure tracing is shown below (Figure 38.1). What is the differential diagnosis?

Restrictive Cardiomyopathy

The pressure tracings show elevated RA pressures with an "M" or "W" sign consistent with impaired diastolic filling. This RA waveform is characteristic of restrictive cardiomyopathy (RCM) and constrictive pericarditis but can be seen in any condition with impaired diastolic filling.

The patient underwent a cardiac MRI (magnetic resonance imaging) that revealed delayed enhancement suggestive of cardiac amyloid. A transmyocardial biopsy was performed approximately a week after the cardiac MRI which confirmed the diagnosis.

RCM is a disease of the myocardium characterized by impaired relaxation and diastolic dysfunction of either or both ventricles. The disease is progressive and as the ventricles become less distensible, diastolic filling and cardiac output are impaired and filling pressures increase. A reduction in systolic function may also occur as the disease progresses. Initial symptoms are usually low output-type complaints (e.g. exertional dyspnea or exercise intolerance) because of inability to augment stroke volume. As RA pressures increases, symptoms of systemic venous congestion may predominate. Further increases in RA and pulmonary capillary wedge (PCW) pressures will be accompanied by symptoms of orthopnea and paroxysmal nocturnal dyspnea. The clinical presentation of RCM can be similar to constrictive pericarditis and differentiation of these processes can be difficult. Additionally, some disease processes (e.g. amyloid, radiation therapy) can involve both myocardium and pericardium, leading to a mixed hemodynamic profile.

A variety of disease states have been identified as causes of RCM that can be broken down into four main categories: noninfiltrative, infiltrative, endomyocardial, and storage diseases. Approximately 50% of cases of RCM have an idiopathic cause; of those in which an etiology is identified, amyloid is the most common diagnosis.

The most common noninfiltrative cause of RCM is idiopathic RCM. This condition is associated with patchy endomyocardial fibrosis, increased cardiac mass, and enlarged atria. It is most commonly seen in older adults, but it may also be seen in children. A clear familial component is present in certain cases of idiopathic RCM, such as in cases also involving Noonan's syndrome.

Infiltrative causes of RCM include amyloidosis, which is the deposition of twisted beta-pleated sheets of fibrils, and sarcoidosis, which is a granulomatous disease of unknown cause. Of the two, amyloidosis is by far the more common cause. There are both genetic and acquired causes of amyloidosis and multiple types of amyloidosis, including primary amyloidosis, secondary amyloidosis, familial amyloidosis, and senile systemic amyloidosis, with each type stemming from a different etiology. Patients with cardiac amyloid will typically present with severe diastolic dysfunction and predominantly right-sided heart failure. Later in the course of disease, patients may also develop loss of left ventricular (LV) systolic function and pulmonary congestion. As amyloid deposits accumulate in the atria, thickening of the interatrial septum and loss of atrial function may also be seen.

Endomyocardial causes of RCM include endomyocardial fibrosis, radiation fibrosis, and anthracycline toxicity. For endomyocardial fibrosis, fibrous endocardial lesions are often seen in the ventricular inflow tracts and frequently involve the atrioventricular (AV) valves, resulting in RCM. As for radiation therapy, it is believed that radiation may cause long-lasting injury to the capillary endothelial cells, resulting in cell death, capillary rupture, and microthrombi, all of which may eventually lead to RCM many years later.

Finally, anthracycline exposure is believed to cause cytotoxicity due to inhibiting an enzyme necessary for DNA repair and generating free radicals that damage cell membranes.

An uncommon cause of RCM is storage disease. An example of a storage disease that causes RCM is hemochromatosis, which is characterized by iron deposition in many organs, including the heart.

Diagnosis and Management

The hemodynamic changes of RCM are similar to those of constrictive pericarditis. There is rapid filling of the ventricles early in diastole, due to high atrial pressures, followed by a phase of minimal passive ventricular filling (due to the stiff myocardium) and then a small amount of additional filling during atrial contraction. Rapid early diastolic filling leads to a prominent "y" descent on the atrial pressure tracings and a "square root" sign on ventricular pressure tracings. In RCM, the "x" descent is frequently blunted (unlike constrictive pericarditis). Increased venous flow

with inspiration is unable to be accommodated by a noncompliant RV; hence, there are diastolic flow reversals in the hepatic vein with inspiration. LV and RV pressures are not interdependent because there is no discordance of intracardiac and intrathoracic pressures (unlike constrictive pericarditis).

On physical examination, RCM often have a prominent apical impulse, S3 and S4, and regurgitant AV valve murmurs. A Kussmaul's sign may be present due to impaired diastolic filling. Paradoxical pulse is typically absent. ECG will commonly exhibit low voltage and may also show atrial enlargement, interventricular conduction delays, and atrial fibrillation. On chest x-ray, an enlarged atria and pulmonary edema may be seen.

Echocardiography is very useful in RCM and often shows diffuse ventricular hypertrophy, small ventricular cavities, and enlarged atria. Increased wall thickness and impaired septal movement with inspiration are other common findings. There is occasionally a "speckling" appearance of the myocardium in cardiac amyloidosis. Doppler imaging reveals a restrictive pattern in a transmitral tracing, with an abnormally high E/A ratio, indicating accentuated early filling

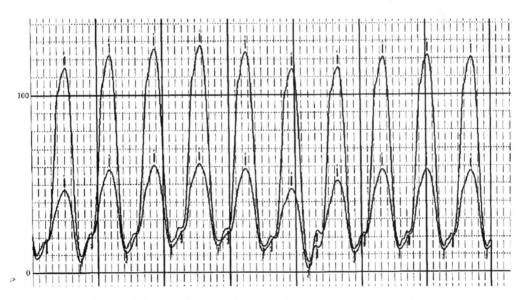

Figure 38.2 Simultaneous left ventricular and right ventricular pressures in a patient with restrictive cardiomyopathy (RCM). Note the similar right ventricular (RV) and left ventricular (LV) diastolic pressure and respiratory concordance.

with diminished late filling. Echocardiographic strain imaging which measures deformation of the myocardium on contraction will often be abnormal prior to development of ventricular hypertrophy.

Cardiac catheterization is an important diagnostic modality. Findings in patients with RCM include pulmonary hypertension, LV end-diastolic pressure (LVEDP) minus RV end-diastolic pressure (RVEDP) greater than 5 mmHg, similar RV and LV diastolic pressures and RA and LV diastolic pressure, and RVEDP less than a third of RV systolic pressure. LV and RV systolic pressures in RCM are concordant during the respiratory cycle, which means they rise and fall in synchrony (Figure 38.2). This is different from constrictive pericarditis where RV and LV systolic pressures are discordant, which means there will be heartbeats in which RV systolic pressure will rise while LV systolic pressure falls (or vice versa) during the respiratory cycle. There is a characteristic "W" sign seen in the RA tracing of patients with RCM.

Cardiac Magnetic Resonance can support the diagnosis of RCM by identifying structural changes in the cardiac chambers. It is also able to facilitate the diagnosis of amyloidosis via a characteristic late gadolinium enhancement pattern. Endomyocardial biopsy is occasionally used to diagnose the cause of RCM.

Further Reading

Garcia, M.J. (2016). Constrictive pericarditis versus restrictive cardiomyopathy? *Journal of the American College of Cardiology* 67 (17): 2061–2076.

Muchtar, E., Blauwet, L.A., and Gertz, M.A. (2017). Restrictive cardiomyopathy: genetics, pathogenesis, clinical manifestations, diagnosis, and therapy. *Circulation Research* 121 (7): 819–837.

McLaughlin, D.P. and Stouffer, G.A. (2017). Restrictive Cardiomyopathy. In: Cardiovascular Hemodynamics for the Clinician, 2e (ed. G. Stouffer), 212–219. Wiley Blackwell. John Wiley & Sons

Case 39: A 66-Year-Old Woman with Chest Pain During a Hurricane

You are asked to see a 66-year-old female with past medical history of thyroid cancer who was brought to the Emergency Department (ED) by Emergency Medical Services after a tree came down in her yard, due to high winds from a hurricane, and crashed through her roof. A branch hit her in the head, causing her to fall to the ground, but she did not lose consciousness. During the ambulance ride and for about an hour after arrival to the ED, she had chest tightness without radiation, nausea, vomiting, or dyspnea. Initial troponin was mildly elevated and increased two hours later.

She denies any cardiac history or any antecedent chest pain symptoms before she was struck by the tree branch. On examination, blood pressure is 132/86 mmHg, heart rate is 96 bpm, and oxygen saturation is 98% on room air. The cardiopulmonary examination is normal. Initial ECG (Figure 39.1), coronary angiography (Figures 39.2 and 39.3), and left ventriculogram (Figure 39.4) are shown below. What is the diagnosis for this patient?

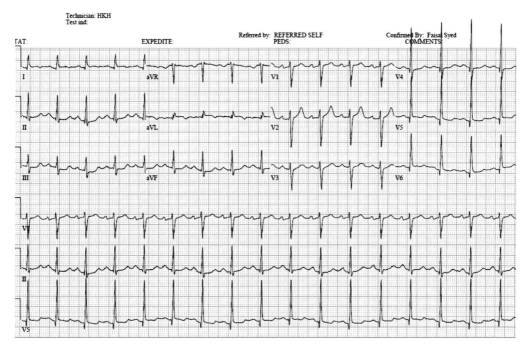

Figure 39.1 ECG on presentation.

Cardiology Board Review: ECG, Hemodynamic and Angiographic Unknowns, First Edition. Edited by George A. Stouffer.
© 2019 John Wiley & Sons Ltd. Published 2019 by John Wiley & Sons Ltd.

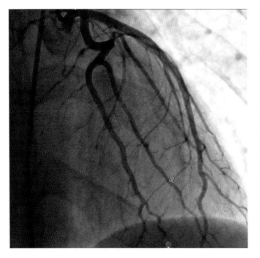 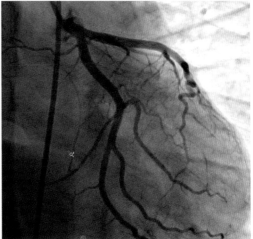

Figure 39.2 Left coronary angiography in an AP (anteroposterior) cranial view and an RAO (right anterior oblique) caudal view.

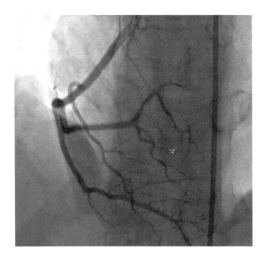

Figure 39.3 Right coronary angiography in an AP cranial view.

Stress-induced Cardiomyopathy

The two most likely diagnoses in this patient include takotsubo cardiomyopathy and non-ST elevation myocardial infarction. Given the lack of coronary artery disease on angiography and the characteristic left ventriculogram, the diagnosis is takotsubo cardiomyopathy, also known as stress-induced cardiomyopathy or broken heart syndrome. This syndrome is characterized by transient systolic dysfunction of the left ventricle, elevated troponins, and an absence of coronary artery disease. The in-hospital mortality rate is approximately 4%, but most patients who survive an acute episode of takotsubo will completely recover within four weeks.

The etiology and pathogenesis of takotsubo cardiomyopathy are not well understood. However, a variety of different clinical situations have been associated with the condition. For example, observational studies have shown that the majority of cases involving takotsubo cardiomyopathy are preceded by either emotional (14–38%) or physiologic (15–77%) stress. As a result, it has been suggested that stress-related mediators, such as excess catecholamines, cytokines, and histamines, could result in coronary artery spasm, microvascular dysfunction, or direct myocardial depressant effects. Any combination of these effects could produce the transient ECG changes, depressed left ventricular function, and elevated cardiac biomarkers that characterize takotsubo cardiomyopathy.

The onset of takotsubo cardiomyopathy begins with a stress-related trigger in approximately 75% of patients. Examples of common stress-related triggers include unexpected death of a loved one, domestic abuse, and devastating financial losses. The classic signs

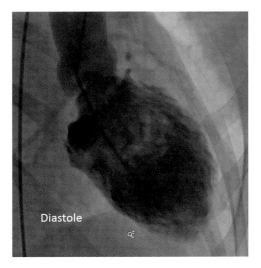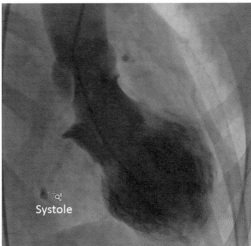

Figure 39.4 Left ventriculography during diastole and systole.

and symptoms of takotsubo include acute substernal chest pain and dyspnea, which can be accompanied by syncope. Heart failure, tachyarrhythmias, bradyarrhythmias, and sudden cardiac death are other findings that may be seen with takotsubo cardiomyopathy.

Electrocardiogram abnormalities usually include ST segment elevations, but can also include abnormal Q waves, ST depressions, and/or T wave inversions. Laboratory findings in takotsubo cardiomyopathy include elevated serum cardiac troponins and elevated BNP (B-type natriuretic peptide). Since most patients with takotsubo cardiomyopathy have high-risk ACS (acute coronary syndrome) features, coronary angiography is often used to define the coronary anatomy.

The diagnosis of takotsubo cardiomyopathy is made based on criteria that were developed at the Mayo Clinic. If all four of Mayo Clinic's criteria are met, then the diagnosis of takotsubo cardiomyopathy can be decisively made:

1) Transient akinesis or dyskinesis of the LV (left ventricular) apical or midventricular segments;
2) Absence of obstructive coronary disease;
3) New ECG abnormalities;
4) Absence of pheochromocytoma and myocarditis.

There are limited data available on treatment for takotsubo cardiomyopathy. However, based on observations from prospective and retrospective case series, current guidelines recommend comparable treatment to that used for patients with cardiomyopathy and systolic dysfunction. This includes a β-blocker, an angiotensin-converting enzyme inhibitor, aspirin, and diuretics, as needed. Until left ventricular function improves, anticoagulation to prevent thrombosis from significant left ventricular dysfunction should also be considered. Patients must be carefully followed to monitor for atrial and ventricular arrhythmias, heart failure, and mechanical complications.

Further Reading

Abe, Y., Kondo, M., Matsuoka, R. et al. (2003). Assessment of clinical features in transient left ventricular apical ballooning. *Journal of the American College of Cardiology* 41 (5): 737–742.

Akashi, Y.J., Goldstein, D.S., Barbaro, G. et al. (2008). Takotsubo cardiomyopathy: a new form of acute, reversible heart failure. *Circulation* 118 (25): 2754–2762.

Bybee, K.A., Kara, T., Prasad, A. et al. (2004a). Systematic review: transient left ventricular apical ballooning: a syndrome that mimics ST-segment elevation myocardial infarction. *Annals of Internal Medicine* 141 (11): 858–865.

Bybee, K.A., Prasad, A., Barsness, G.W. et al. (2004b). Clinical characteristics and thrombolysis in myocardial infarction frame counts in women with transient left ventricular apical ballooning syndrome. *The American Journal of Cardiology* 94 (3): 343–346. https://doi.org/10.1016/j. amjcard.2004.04.030.

Chiles, C.D., Patel, R. and Baggett, C. (2019). Stress-induced cardiomyopathy. In: *Netter's Cardiology*, 3e (ed. G. Stouffer, M. Runge, C. Patterson and J.S. Rossi). Elsevier.

Desmet, W.J.R., Adriaenssens, B.F.M., and Dens, J.A.Y. (2003). Apical ballooning of the left ventricle: first series in white patients. *Heart* 89 (9): 1027–1031.

Krishnamoorthy, P., Garg, J., Sharma, A. et al. (2015). Gender differences and predictors of mortality in Takotsubo cardiomyopathy: analysis from the National Inpatient Sample 2009–2010 database. *Cardiology* 132 (2): 131–136. https://doi.org/10.1159/ 000430782.

Ogura, R., Hiasa, Y., Takahashi, T. et al. (2003). Specific findings of the standard 12-lead ECG in patients with "Takotsubo" cardiomyopathy: comparison with the findings of acute anterior myocardial infarction. *Circulation Journal* 67 (8): 687–690.

Sharkey, S.W., Lesser, J.R., Zenovich, A.G. et al. (2005). Acute and reversible cardiomyopathy provoked by stress in women from the United States. *Circulation* 111 (4): 472–479.

Templin, C., Ghadri, J.R., Diekmann, J. et al. (2015). Clinical features and outcomes of Takotsubo (stress) cardiomyopathy. *The New England Journal of Medicine* 373 (10): 929–938. https://doi.org/10.1056/ NEJMoa1406761.

Tsuchihashi, K., Ueshima, K., Uchida, T. et al. (2001). Transient left ventricular apical ballooning without coronary artery stenosis: a novel heart syndrome mimicking acute myocardial infarction. Angina pectoris-myocardial infarction investigations in Japan. *Journal of the American College of Cardiology* 38 (1): 11–18.

Watanabe, H., Kodama, M., Okura, Y. et al. (2005). Impact of earthquakes on Takotsubo cardiomyopathy. *Journal of the American Medical Association* 294 (3): 305–307. https://doi.org/10.1001/ jama.294.3.305.

Wittstein, I.S., Thiemann, D.R., Lima, J.A.C. et al. (2005). Neurohumoral features of myocardial stunning due to sudden emotional stress. *The New England Journal of Medicine* 352 (6): 539–548. https://doi. org/10.1056/NEJMoa043046.

Case 40: A 39-Year-Old Woman Who is Found Unconscious

A 39-year-old female is brought to the Emergency Department with abrupt onset of altered state of consciousness. She is a known illicit drug user with her most recent drug of choice being cocaine. Past medical history includes end-stage renal disease on hemodialysis, long-standing severe hypertension, and a history of pulmonary embolism.

The Emergency Department physician asks your opinion about the ECG and specifically wants to know whether you think the patient is having myocardial ischemia. The current ECG (Figure 40.1a) has changed compared to an ECG from one month ago (Figure 40.1b). Is this patient having myocardial ischemia and what clues does the ECG provide in establishing a differential diagnosis of the altered state of consciousness?

Intracerebral Bleed

The current ECG shows sinus rhythm with prolonged QTc interval, pseudonormalization of T waves in the lateral leads, biphasic T waves in the anterior leads, and diffuse T wave flattening in the other leads. ECG one month prior (Figure 40.1b) showed normal sinus regular rhythm at a rate of 84 beats per minute. P wave and QRS duration and axis are within normal limits. There is T wave inversion in leads I and aVL and the patient may have left ventricular hypertrophy (LVH) by the Cornell voltage criteria (S in V3 + R in aVL >20 mm). Comparison of the two ECGs shows that major changes include prolongation of the QTc interval and diffuse T wave changes. These changes are nonspecific, however the pattern of a marked increase in the QTc interval and diffuse ST/T wave changes, in a patient with altered mental status, should prompt consideration of the diagnosis of an intracerebral event. In this patient, a head CT showed basal ganglia hemorrhage with hydrocephalus.

Acute brain injury, via hemorrhage, trauma, meningitis, malignancy, or other causes, can result in ECG changes and arrhythmias and in rare cases, cardiac dysfunction and isoenzyme elevation. The majority of patients with intracerebral hemorrhage present with ECG abnormalities such as prolonged QT intervals, ST segment elevation or depression, inverted T waves, and/or ventricular ectopy. ST segment elevation mimicking acute infarction and acute pericarditis has been described. The ECG changes are dynamic and may evolve over several days. The mechanism has not been clearly established but is thought to relate to an abrupt elevation of serum catecholamine levels with or without decreased parasympathetic nervous activity. Intracerebral hemorrhage also has effects on intracellular Ca^{2+} regulation of cardiac myocytes.

Occasionally, the ECG can provide clues that are helpful in the diagnosis of rare causes of altered mental status. A short QTc interval is found in severe hypercalcemia. Sinus bradycardia and low voltage are seen in hypothyroidism. QRS widening, especially in the

Cardiology Board Review: ECG, Hemodynamic and Angiographic Unknowns, First Edition. Edited by George A. Stouffer.
© 2019 John Wiley & Sons Ltd. Published 2019 by John Wiley & Sons Ltd.

(a) - ECG on presentation

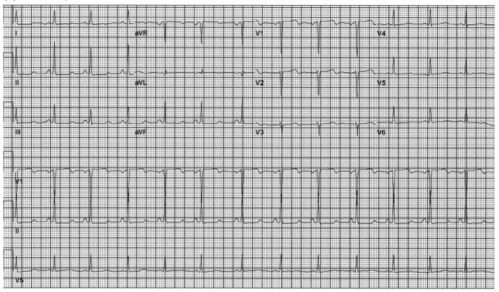

(b) - ECG one month previously

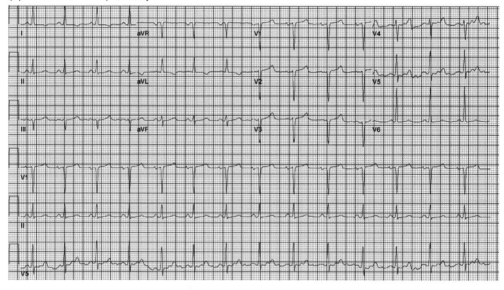

Figure 40.1 ECG while patient is in Emergency Department (a) and one month previously (b).

presence of QTc prolongation, is consistent with an overdose of tricyclic antidepressants.

Ischemic changes can suggest carbon monoxide poisoning.

Further Reading

van Bree, M.D.R., Roos, Y.B., van der Bilt, I.A.C. et al. (2010). Prevalence and characterization of ECG abnormalities after intracerebral hemorrhage. *Neurocritical Care* 12 (1): 50–55.

Qaqa, A.Y., Suleiman, A., Alsumrain, M. et al. (2012). Electrocardiographic abnormalities in patients presenting with intracranial parenchymal haemorrhage. *Acta Cardiologica* 67 (6): 635–639.

Case 41: An Unusual Right Atrial Pressure Tracing

You are performing a right heart catheterization on a 67-year-old female with exertional dyspnea and obtain the following right atrial pressure tracing (Figure 41.1). What is the diagnosis?

Severe Tricuspid Regurgitation

The normal right atrium (RA) waveform consists of an A wave associated with atrial contraction, a C wave associated with ventricular

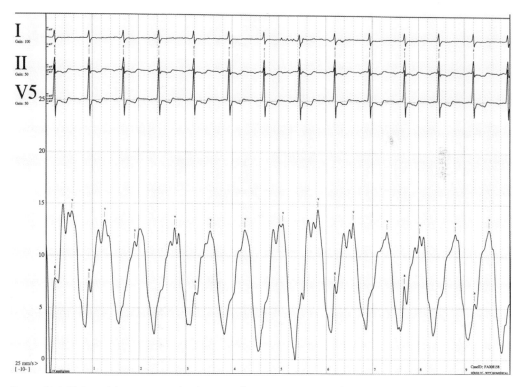

Figure 41.1 Right atrial pressure tracing (measured on a 0–25 mmHg scale).

Cardiology Board Review: ECG, Hemodynamic and Angiographic Unknowns, First Edition. Edited by George A. Stouffer.
© 2019 John Wiley & Sons Ltd. Published 2019 by John Wiley & Sons Ltd.

contraction, and a V wave associated with rising atrial pressure just prior to opening of the tricuspid valve. With volumetrically important tricuspid regurgitation, there is a large systolic wave in the right atrial tracing reflecting retrograde ejection of blood and consequent transmission of pressure from the right ventricle (RV) to the RA. This waveform is variously termed an S wave or a CV wave as it occurs during systole and subsumes the normally independent C and V waves. The magnitude of the systolic wave is determined both by the severity of the regurgitation, and the compliance of the RA.

In patients with severe tricuspid regurgitation, the systolic wave in the RA becomes so prominent that the tracing resembles the right ventricular tracing (Figure 41.1). In very severe tricuspid regurgitation the RA and RV pressure tracings are virtually identical, reflecting the fact that in the absence of a competent tricuspid valve, the RA and RV become, functionally, a single chamber.

This was evident in this patient during simultaneous recording of RA and RV pressures (Figure 41.2).

Tricuspid regurgitation can be classified as primary or secondary (functional). Primary tricuspid valve structural abnormalities are rare, but can be due to rheumatic heart disease, myxomatous disease (prolapse), infective or marantic endocarditis, carcinoid heart disease, anorectic drugs, trauma, Marfan's syndrome, or Ebstein's anomaly. The tricuspid valve can also be damaged during placement of leads for pacemakers or implantable cardioverter-defibrillators or during right ventricular biopsies in heart transplant recipients.

Secondary functional tricuspid regurgitation is commonly encountered as a consequence of conditions associated with increased pulmonary arterial pressures such as left ventricular systolic or diastolic dysfunction, mitral regurgitation, mitral stenosis, primary pulmonary disease, or primary pulmonary hypertension. Dilatation of the

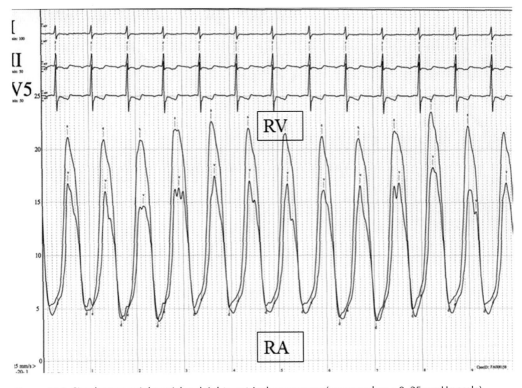

Figure 41.2 Simultaneous right atrial and right ventricular pressures (measured on a 0–25 mmHg scale).

tricuspid annulus may also be seen in right ventricular infarction or in dilated cardio-myopathies. Echocardiography can estimate the severity of tricuspid regurgitation and also provide information about the mechanism.

Further Reading

Andersen, M.J., Nishimura, R.A., and Borlaug, B.A. (2014). The hemodynamic basis of exercise intolerance in tricuspid regurgitation. *Circulation: Heart Failure* 7 (6): 911–917.

Baumgartner, H., Falk, V., Bax, J.J. et al. (2017). 2017 ESC/EACTS guidelines for the management of valvular heart disease. *European Heart Journal* 38: 2739–2791.

Nishimura, R.A., Otto, C.M., Bonow, R.O. et al. (2014). 2014 AHA/ACC guideline for the management of patients with valvular heart disease: a report of the American College of Cardiology/American Heart Association Task Force on Practice Guidelines. *Journal of the American College of Cardiology* 63 (22): e57–e185.

Rao, S., Tate, D.A., and Stouffer, G.A. (2013). Hemodynamic findings in severe tricuspid regurgitation. *Catheterization and Cardiovascular Interventions* 81(1): 162–169.

Case 42: A 20-Year-Old Man with a Heart Rate of 250 bpm

You are making rounds on the Cardiology Service when you receive a stat page to come to the Emergency Department. A 20-year-old male was brought in by Emergency Medical Services a few minutes previously complaining of palpitations and not feeling well. Upon questioning, he reports using cocaine at the onset of symptoms.

On physical examination, he is ill-appearing and sweating profusely. Blood pressure is 80 mmHg systolic and heart rate is approximately 250 bpm. You ask for an ECG which is shown below (Figure 42.1).

After Cardioversion

The ECG shows an irregular wide complex tachycardia. The differential diagnosis includes atrial fibrillation with conduction via an accessory pathway or polymorphic ventricular tachycardia. In a rhythm this

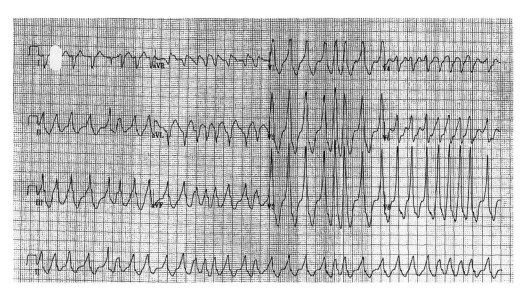

Figure 42.1 ECG at presentation.

Cardiology Board Review: ECG, Hemodynamic and Angiographic Unknowns, First Edition. Edited by George A. Stouffer.
© 2019 John Wiley & Sons Ltd. Published 2019 by John Wiley & Sons Ltd.

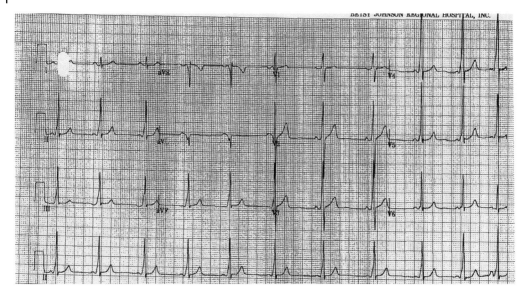

Figure 42.2 ECG after cardioversion.

irregular, atrial fibrillation with aberrancy is the most common mechanism. Because of worries about hemodynamic deterioration with pharmacological treatment, the patient is electrically cardioverted. The ECG after cardioversion is shown above (Figure 42.2). What is the diagnosis?

Atrial Fibrillation with Wolff–Parkinson–White Syndrome

The initial ECG shows an irregular wide complex tachycardia. The degree of irregularity is consistent with atrial fibrillation and the wide complex nature suggests aberrant atrioventricular (AV) conduction. The ECG following cardioversion shows a pattern of pre-excitation which means that electrical impulses from the atrium to the ventricle are being conducted via one or more accessory pathways rather than via the AV node. An accessory pathway (also known as a bypass tract) is a thin filamentous structure that has conductive properties and thus enables the electrical impulse to go from the atria to the ventricles without passing through the AV

node. While numerous locations of accessory pathways have been reported including atriofascicular, fasciculoventricular, intranodal, or nodoventricular, the most common bypass tract is a direct connection between the atria and ventricles and is known as a Kent bundle. Accessory pathways, in general, do not have decremental conduction (defined as rate dependent prolongation of conduction time) and thus do not have the normal safety mechanisms of the AV node in controlling ventricular rates.

ECG findings of pre-excitation include a short PR interval (0.12 seconds; because conduction down the accessory pathway is faster than through the AV node; Figure 42.3), widening of the QRS complex (>0.12 seconds) and delta waves (slurred, slow-rising onset of QRS seen best in the inferior leads and in leads V1 → V4 in this case). Less commonly, repolarization abnormalities (e.g. T wave inversions) will also be present. The PR interval, the time required for the atria to depolarize, and the wave of depolarisation to arrive at the ventricles is shortened in pre-excitation syndromes because the accessory pathway permits the impulse to bypass the AV node. A portion of the ventricles (depending on where the accessory pathway

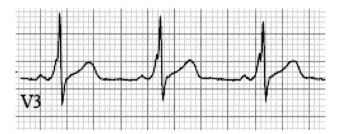

Figure 42.3 ECG tracing showing short PR interval and delta wave.

inserts) activates first, leading to an initial slurring or "delta wave" at the start of the QRS complex. Conduction also occurs via the AV node and thus simultaneous activation of both ventricles can occur via the His-Purkinje system. Thus the size of the delta wave and the QRS duration is a function of where in the ventricles the accessory pathway inserts and the amount of relative conduction between the accessory pathway and the AV node.

Accessory pathways are congenital in origin and result from a failure of complete separation of the atria and ventricles. Approximately 0.1–0.3% of the general population have ECG findings of pre-excitation. The incidence of associated congenital abnormalities (e.g. Ebstein's anomaly, atrial septal defect, ventricular septal defect, tricuspid atresia, aortic coarctation) ranges from 7 to 20%. In around 10% of cases multiple accessory pathways exist.

Subjects with ventricular pre-excitation on the ECG but who are asymptomatic and have no clinical arrhythmias are usually described as having "ventricular pre-excitation" or "a Wolff–Parkinson–White (WPW) ECG pattern." When arrhythmias are present, the disorder is called the WPW syndrome. A concealed pathway is said to be present if the accessory pathway only conducts retrograde. In this case, the resting ECG will be normal in sinus rhythm with no evidence of pre-excitation.

The most frequently encountered arrhythmias in WPW (in order of occurrence) are: (i) orthodromic atrioventricular reentrant tachycardia (AVRT); (ii) atrial fibrillation; and (iii) antidromic AVRT. The AVRT arrhythmias are due to a reentry circuit that involves the AV node and the accessory pathway(s) and are generally triggered by an atrial ectopic beat. Orthodromic AVRT involves antegrade conduction down the AV node (with retrograde conduction via the accessory pathway) and results in a narrow complex tachycardia since the ventricles are activated via the normal conduction system (the delta wave will disappear during this arrhythmia). In can be difficult to definitively diagnose orthodromic AVRT during an episode of narrow complex tachycardia but clues include a rate that is usually between 140 and 250 beats per minute and inverted P waves within the ST segment, indicating that atrial depolarization is occurring after ventricular depolarisation. Orthodromic AVRTs account for most tachycardias in WPW syndrome. Antidromic tachycardias occur when the ventricles are activated via the accessory pathway (i.e. antegrade conduction in the accessory pathway and retrograde conduction in the AV node). This results in a wide QRS reflecting abnormal ventricular activation (Figure 42.4).

For reasons that are not clear atrial fibrillation is more common in WPW syndrome than in the normal population. In atrial fibrillation, activation of the ventricles is predominantly via the accessory pathway which causes an irregular wide complex tachycardia as observed in this case. Atrial fibrillation can be life-threatening if the accessory pathway has a short anterograde refractory period, allowing rapid conduction of the atrial impulses to the ventricle. This will

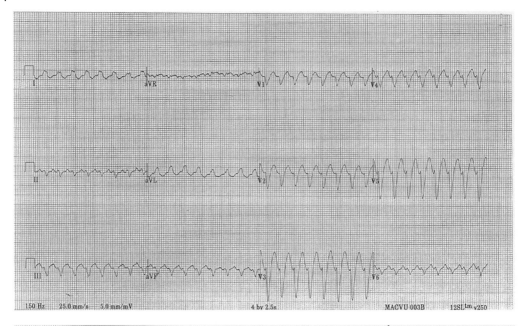

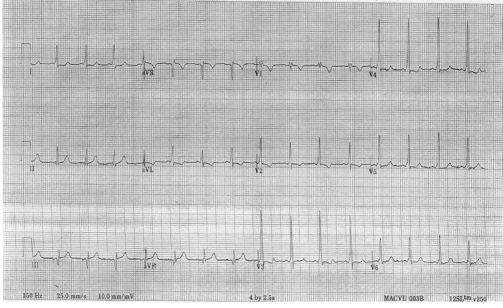

Figure 42.4 ECG in a 38-year-old male with Wolff–Parkinson–White (WPW) syndrome during an antidromic tachycardia and after conversion to sinus rhythm.

result in very high ventricular rates with possible deterioration into ventricular fibrillation and sudden death.

The location of the accessory pathway can be approximated based on the 12 lead ECG. In type A, the QRS complex is positive in V1 and V2 and this correlates with a left-side accessory pathway (a posteroseptal location characterized by a leftward axis and a lateral pathway characterized by an inferior axis). In the more common type B, the QRS complex is negative in V1 and V2.

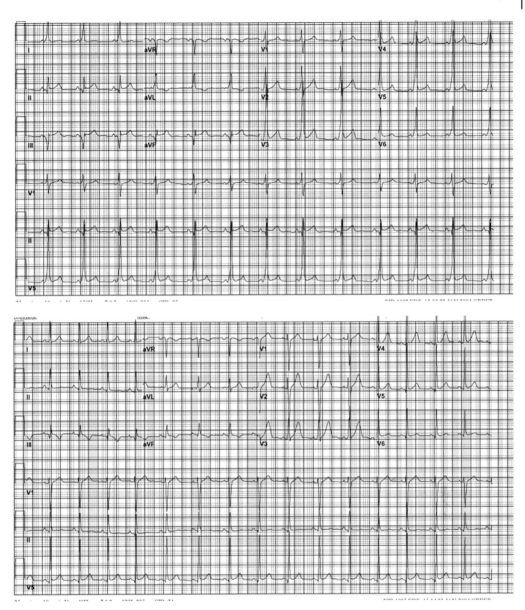

Figure 42.5 ECG of a patient with Wolff–Parkinson–White (WPW) before and after catheter ablation of an accessory pathway.

This correlates with a right-sided pathway (posteroseptal and lateral pathways have a leftward axis while an anteroseptal pathway is negative in both V1 and V2 with a normal axis). Type A is occasionally confused with a right bundle branch block (RBBB), right ventricular hypertrophy (RVH), or an inferior myocardial infarction (MI), while type

B can be confused with left bundle branch block (LBBB) or anterior MI. This patient had a type A pathway.

If a patient is symptomatic, treatment can be either pharmacological or by catheter ablation. Elimination of an accessory pathway by catheter ablation can be curative and result in normalization of the ECG

(Figure 42.5). Treatment of asymptomatic individuals to prevent sudden cardiac death is controversial and the reader is directed to the extensive literature on this subject for a more complete discussion.

There is a rare syndrome, Lown–Ganong–Levine (LGL), which is characterized by a short PR but a normal QRS. In this syndrome, there is an accessory pathway (James fibers) that connects directly with the His bundle. A note of caution is that not all patients with short PR intervals and normal QRS complexes have LGL as there are other causes of this combination.

Further Reading

Al-Khatib, S.M., Arshad, A., Balk, E.M. et al. (2016). Risk stratification for arrhythmic events in patients with asymptomatic pre-excitation: a systematic review for the 2015 ACC/AHA/HRS guideline for the management of adult patients with supraventricular tachycardia: a report of the American College of Cardiology/American Heart Association Task Force on Clinical Practice Guidelines and the Heart Rhythm Society. *Journal of the American College of Cardiology* 67 (13): 1624–1638.

Page, R.L., Joglar, J.A., Caldwell, M.A. et al. (2016). 2015 ACC/AHA/HRS guideline for the management of adult patients with supraventricular tachycardia: a report of the American College of Cardiology/American Heart Association Task Force on Clinical Practice Guidelines and the Heart Rhythm Society. *Journal of the American College of Cardiology* 67 (13): e27–e115.

Tracy, C.M., Epstein, A.E., Darbar, D. et al. (2013). 2012 ACCF/AHA/HRS focused update incorporated into the ACCF/AHA/HRS 2008 guidelines for device-based therapy of cardiac rhythm abnormalities: a report of the American College of Cardiology Foundation/American Heart Association Task Force on Practice Guidelines and the Heart Rhythm Society. *Journal of the American College of Cardiology* 61 (3): e6–e75.

Case 43: A 46-Year-Old Man with Heart Failure and New Onset Palpitations

You are asked to see a 46-year-old male with ischemic cardiomyopathy (ejection fraction of 25%) and atrial fibrillation who presented to the Emergency Department with complaints of palpitations for approximately 12 hours. He reports nausea and vomiting for several days which has recently worsened. He has continued to take his current mediations which include metoprolol, digoxin, benazepril, atorvastatin, aspirin, and furosemide.

Physical examination is remarkable for a blood pressure of 85/62 mmHg, pulse rate of 110 bpm, and oxygen saturation of 93% on room air. His lungs have crackles at the base and he has a soft systolic murmur along the left upper sternal border. There is 2+ edema at the ankles.

What clues does the ECG provide in establishing a differential diagnosis (Figure 43.1)?

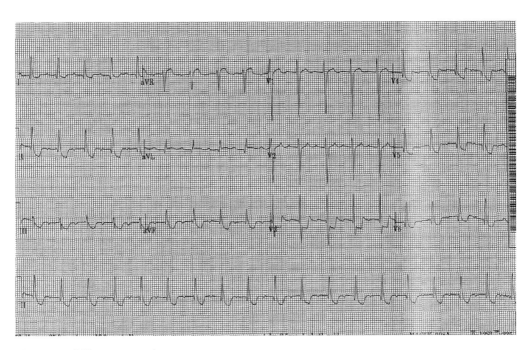

Figure 43.1 ECG on presentation.

Cardiology Board Review: ECG, Hemodynamic and Angiographic Unknowns, First Edition. Edited by George A. Stouffer.
© 2019 John Wiley & Sons Ltd. Published 2019 by John Wiley & Sons Ltd.

Digoxin Toxicity

This ECG shows a regular, narrow complex tachycardia at a rate of approximately 140 bpm. There are P waves prior to each QRS complex with a prolonged PR interval. The P wave axis is abnormal (negative in II, III, and aVF) and thus the rhythm is an atrial tachycardia with first-degree atrioventricular (AV) block. The QT interval is short and there are pronounced diffuse ST abnormalities. The combination of an atrial tachycardia with AV block, shortened QT interval, and diffuse ST changes is consistent with a diagnosis of digoxin toxicity. This patient's digoxin level was 8 nmol/l (therapeutic concentration is generally 1–2 nmol/l). He was given Digibind, a specific antidote for digoxin toxicity which utilizes antigen-binding fragments (Fab) derived from specific anti-digoxin antibodies raised in sheep to neutralize circulating digoxin. After treatment, ECG showed sinus rhythm (note that the P wave axis has normalized) with a rate of approximately 84 bpm and resolution of ST segment depression (Figure 43.2).

Digitalis derivatives are found in several plants, including oleander and foxglove (*Digitalis lanata*), and are used therapeutically as digoxin or digitoxin. Cardiac glycosides have both inotropic and AV blocking effects and were once widely used in heart failure and atrial fibrillation. They are now less popular but occasionally still utilized in selected patients.

The effects of digitalis result from the inhibition of the sodium-potassium adenosine triphosphatase (NA^+/K^+ ATPase) pump. It binds in a reversible process to a specific site on the extracytoplasmic surface of the alpha subunit of the sodium- and potassium-activated adenosine triphosphatase (NaK ATPase) pump. This results in an increase in intracellular sodium and a decrease in intracellular potassium. The increase in intracellular Na^+ levels reduces the extrusion of calcium (Ca^{2+}) by the Na^+/Ca^{2+} exchange pump, resulting in increased intracellular Ca^{2+} which increases the force of myocardial contraction. These effects cause a decreased resting potential which slows the rate of phase 0 depolarization, a decrease in action

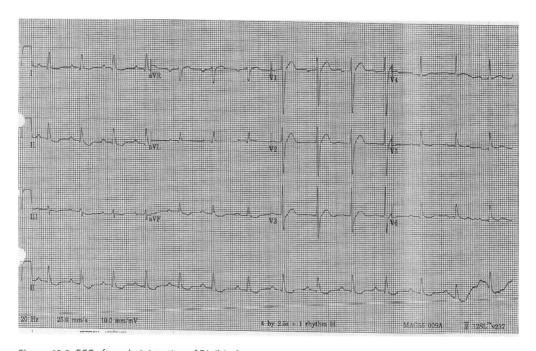

Figure 43.2 ECG after administration of Digibind.

potential duration, and enhanced automaticity which results in an increase in the rate of phase 4 depolarization. Digitalis also has a negative chronotropic action, which is due to increased vagal tone and direct effects on the sinoatrial (SA) and AV nodes.

The effect of digitalis on cardiac cells and thus the potential for toxicity is a function of various factors including amount ingested, renal excretion (which is regulated by renal function, dehydration, drug interactions, etc), and electrolyte levels. Hypokalemia, hypernatremia, or hypomagnesemia increase the toxic cardiovascular effects of digitalis because of their depressive effects on the NA^+/K^+ ATPase pump. Acidosis and myocardial ischemia will also affect the response to digitalis. Various medications can affect digitalis levels including antiarrhythmics (e.g. amiodarone, quinidine), diuretics, antibiotics, and cyclosporine.

Digitalis effects on the baseline ECG include a shortened QT, downward sagging or "scooping" of the ST segment with concomitant ST depression (this is usually most pronounced in the lateral leads), an increase in U wave amplitude, and T wave changes. Direct effect of digitalis on repolarization is often reflected in the ECG by ST segment and T wave forces opposite in direction to the predominant QRS force. These findings can occur at therapeutic concentrations and are not indicative of toxicity. In contrast, PR or QRS prolongation, varying degrees of AV block, and arrhythmias may signify digitalis toxicity. Cardiac dysrhythmias associated with digitalis generally arise from either an increase in automaticity or a decrease in conduction. Premature ventricular contractions are the most common arrhythmia associated with digitalis toxicity but other arrhythmias that can be seen include atrial tachycardia, junctional tachycardia, ventricular tachycardia, atrial flutter, alternating ventricular pacemakers, SA arrest, and varying degrees of AV block. Almost any dysrhythmia may be precipitated by digitalis except sinus tachycardia, AV nodal reentrant tachycardia, AV reciprocating tachycardia, and rapid atrial fibrillation. Atrial tachycardia with AV block and bidirectional ventricular tachycardia (alternating bundle branch blocks) are particularly characteristic of severe digitalis toxicity. Although there is no single arrhythmia that is diagnostic of digitalis toxicity, the combination of enhanced automaticity and impaired conduction (e.g. atrial tachycardia with first-degree AV block as in this patient) should raise suspicion of toxicity in a patient treated with digitalis.

Further Reading

Roberts, D.M., Gallapatthy, G., Dunuwille, A. et al. (2016). Pharmacological treatment of cardiac glycoside poisoning. *British Journal of Clinical Pharmacology* 81 (3): 488–495.

Case 44: Palpitations and Dizziness in a Young Adult with a Very Abnormal ECG

A 28-year-old man without past medical history presents to the Emergency Department with complaints of palpitations and dizziness. He denies use of illicit drugs but admits to drinking several "energy drinks" earlier today.

The Emergency Department physician is worried about the ECG and gives you a call. What is your interpretation of the ECG and what do you recommend to the individual (Figure 44.1)?

Apical Hypertrophic Cardiomyopathy

Apical hypertrophic cardiomyopathy (AHCM) is an uncommon variant of hypertrophic cardiomyopathy (HCM) that was initially described in Japan but has since been recognized in many other ethnic groups. AHCM is defined by thickened apical segments which produce a "spade-shaped" small apical cavity.

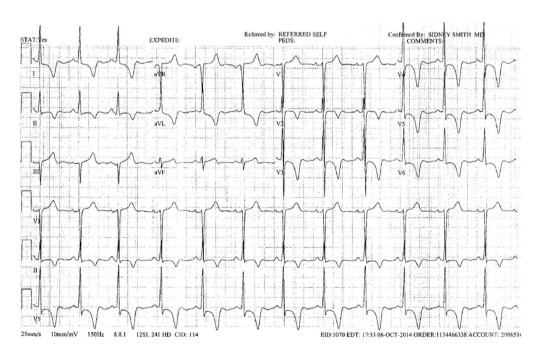

Figure 44.1 ECG on presentation.

Cardiology Board Review: ECG, Hemodynamic and Angiographic Unknowns, First Edition. Edited by George A. Stouffer.
© 2019 John Wiley & Sons Ltd. Published 2019 by John Wiley & Sons Ltd.

The ECG is characterized by pronounced inverted precordial T-waves; other ECG findings include left ventricular hypertrophy (LVH) with deep, inverted T waves in leads I, II, aVL, and V3–V6. It is important to note that giant negative T waves are not invariably seen in AHCM and that the depth of the negative T waves and ST segment depression has been reported to vary over time. ECG findings provide an important clue but AHCM is generally diagnosed by transthoracic echocardiography.

HCM in general is caused by a mutation in one of the gene-encoding proteins of the cardiac sarcomere. At least 10 different genes have been linked to HCM, but three genes predominate: β-myosin heavy chain, cardiac troponin T, and myosin-binding protein C. Familial HCM is an autosomal dominant disease and present in 50% of patients with HCM; spontaneous mutations are suspected for sporadic forms of the disease. The phenotypic expression of HCM occurs in 1 of every 500 adults in the general population and includes ventricular hypertrophy. Different forms of HCM include asymmetrical hypertrophy of the interventricular septum (with or without an outflow tract gradient), concentric hypertrophy, and apical hypertrophy. Hypertrophy can be found in any region of the left ventricle, but it is most frequently found in the septum. Extensive fibrosis of the affected walls occurs as well. Dynamic left ventricular outflow tract obstruction (used to differentiate hypertrophic obstructive cardiomyopathy [HOCM] from the larger group of HCM) is present in 30–50% of patients with HCM.

HCM can present at any age. The majority of patients are asymptomatic throughout life but some patients will develop dyspnea, angina, palpitations, and syncope. Symptoms primarily result from hemodynamic alterations which include dynamic left ventricular outflow tract obstruction, mitral regurgitation, diastolic dysfunction, and myocardial ischemia. The most feared complication of the disease is sudden cardiac death, primarily due to ventricular arrhythmias.

In contrast to AHCM where the ECG can be highly suggestive, there is no characteristic ECG pattern that is diagnostic in the vast majority of HCM (although the 12-lead ECG is abnormal in 75–95% of HCM patients). The most common ECG findings in HCM are due to LVH and include increased voltage and repolarization abnormalities. LVH can cause delayed propagation of impulses in hypertrophied myocardium leading to an increased angle between the QRS and T axes; a wide angle accompanied by increased QRS amplitude is known as left ventricular strain. T wave inversion and ST segment depression with upward convexity is commonly seen in V4–V6, while tall T waves and ST segment elevation are present in the right precordial leads. Because many HCM patients have septal hypertrophy, abnormal Q waves are common. These Q waves commonly mimic those of a myocardial infarction. The increased amplitude of electrical forces from depolarization of the hypertrophied septum can cause deep Q waves in the lateral and inferior leads and taller R waves in the right precordial leads. T wave abnormalities are present in most symptomatic HCM patients. Septal hypertrophy causes the T wave to be directed opposite of prominent septal depolarization force, so the T wave will be positive in leads with a deep Q waves. Left atrial abnormality and prolonged QTc interval can also be seen in patients with obstructive HCM. Atrial fibrillation is the most common sustained arrhythmia in HCM but atrial flutter, ventricular ectopy, ventricular tachycardia, and ventricular fibrillation can also occur. In rare cases, there can be PR prolongation or ECG findings of pre-excitation (Wolff–Parkinson–White pattern).

Further Reading

Maron, B.J. (2018). Clinical course and management of hypertrophic cardiomyopathy. *New England Journal of Medicine* 379 (7): 655–668.

Maron, B.J., Ommen, S.R., Semsarian, C. et al. (2014). Hypertrophic cardiomyopathy: present and future, with translation into contemporary cardiovascular medicine. *Journal of the American College of Cardiology* 64 (1): 83–99.

Zeineh, N.S. and Eles, G. (2015). Apical hypertrophic cardiomyopathy. *New England Journal of Medicine* 373 (19): e22.

Case 45: A 36-Year-Old Man with Long-Standing Hypertension and an Abnormal ECG

A 36-year-old male with severe hypertension and end-stage renal disease is sent to you by his primary care physician because of an abnormal ECG. The patient denies cardiac symptoms and remains active. On physician examination, his blood pressure is 165/105 mmHg, heart rate is 66 bpm, and oxygen saturation is 99% on room air. Current medications include labetolol, amlodipine, and hydralazine. The ECG is shown below (Figure 45.1). What is your interpretation?

Left Ventricular Hypertrophy

Electrical forces generated during left ventricular (LV) activation produce the QRS complex. With an increase in the amount of LV myocardium, electrical preponderance of LV over RV (right ventricle) is further accentuated. The mean vector of the LV becomes more posterior and leftward, increasing QRS complex voltage and ventricular activation time. Additional ECG clues to the diagnosis

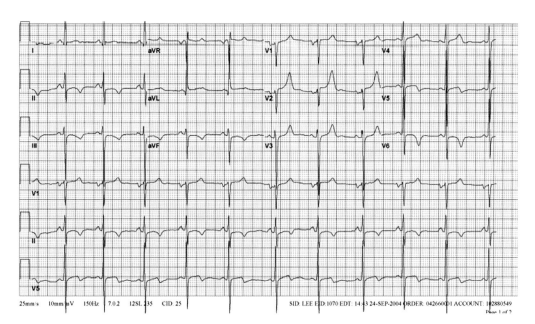

Figure 45.1 ECG on presentation.

Cardiology Board Review: ECG, Hemodynamic and Angiographic Unknowns, First Edition. Edited by George A. Stouffer.
© 2019 John Wiley & Sons Ltd. Published 2019 by John Wiley & Sons Ltd.

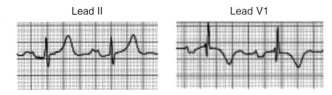

Lead II   Lead V1

Figure 45.2 An example of left atrial abnormality (LAA).

of LVH (left ventricular hypertrophy) are left axis deviation, increased QRS duration, ST-T abnormalities (a "strain pattern"), and the presence of left atrial abnormality (LAA) (Figure 45.2).

There are numerous published criteria that can be used to diagnose LVH on an ECG, although none is universally accepted. Some of these criteria are based solely on voltage present on the ECG (e.g. the Sokolow-Lyon Voltage Criteria and the Cornell Voltage Criteria), whereas others also take into account related findings such as left axis deviation, LAA, and ST-T wave abnormalities (e.g. the Estes Criteria). For all of these formulas, the specificity tends to be high while the sensitivity is much lower. To further complicate the situation, the sensitivity and specificity of the various ECG criteria vary with age, gender, and obesity. Modified formulas that "correct" for these variables have been developed for some of the specific criteria (e.g. Cornell criteria). Despite all of these limitations, the ECG remains a useful, although far from perfect tool to identify ventricular hypertrophy.

On voltage criteria alone, there is general agreement that LVH may be diagnosed based either on increased voltage in the limb leads (R wave in lead I plus S wave in lead III >25 mm or R wave in lead aVL >11 mm or R wave in lead aVF >20 mm) or increased voltage in the precordial leads (S wave in V1 exceeding 24 mm or R wave in leads V4, V5, or V6 > 26 mm or R wave in leads V5 or 6 plus S wave in lead V1 > 35 mm).

LAA is suggested by notching or prominence of the terminal portion of the P wave in the limb leads, prominent negativity of the terminal portion of the P wave in V1, or a P wave duration of >120 ms (Figure 45.2). Normal P waves may be bifid in the limb leads with a minor notch probably resulting from slight asynchrony between right and left atrial depolarisation. However, a pronounced notch with a peak-to-peak interval of >0.04 seconds suggests LAA. In V1, the P wave is often biphasic. This occurs because early right atrial forces are directed anteriorly giving rise to an initial positive deflection, whereas left atrial forces travel posteriorly, producing a later negative deflection. A large negative deflection (>1 small square in area) suggests LAA.

LAA from hypertension must be distinguished from P-mitrale which is defined as a widened P wave (≥0.12 seconds) with normal or slightly increased voltage that is notched, bifid or flat-topped. It is a sign of long-standing mitral valve disease.

Further Reading

Alfakih, K., Walters, K., Jones, T. et al. (2004). New gender-specific partition values for ECG criteria of left ventricular hypertrophy: recalibration against cardiac MRI. *Hypertension* 44 (2): 175–179.

Sundström, J., Lind, L., Ärnlöv, J. et al. (2001). Echocardiographic and electrocardiographic diagnoses of left ventricular hypertrophy predict mortality independently of each other in a population of elderly men. *Circulation* 103 (19): 2346–2351.

Surawicz, B. and Knilans, T. (2008). *Left Ventricular Enlargement in Chou's Electrocardiography in Clinical Practice E-Book: Adult and Pediatric.* Elsevier Health Sciences.

Case 46: A 46-Year-Old Man with Fatigue

A 46-year-old male is referred to you for evaluation of fatigue and a murmur. A murmur was diagnosed approximately five years ago on a routine annual physical examination. He originally had no symptoms but over the last year has become more and more fatigued with his morning workout routine. It has progressed to where he can only exercise for 20 minutes on an elliptical machine, whereas a year ago he could complete 45 minutes. On exam, his heart rate is 75 bpm and blood pressure is 120/80 mmHg. He has a normal S1, a soft S2, and a loud systolic murmur heartbeat at the apex.

After an echocardiogram is obtained, he was referred for cardiac catheterization. A left ventriculogram is shown below (Figure 46.1). What is the diagnosis?

Severe Mitral Regurgitation

The left atrium becomes opacified at the same level as the left ventricle during left ventriculography (Figure 46.2). Prior to cardiac catheterization, he had an echocardiogram which showed severe mitral regurgitation (MR), prolapse of P2, and left ventricular enlargement. Coronary angiography showed no significant coronary disease, and he underwent minimally invasive mitral valve repair.

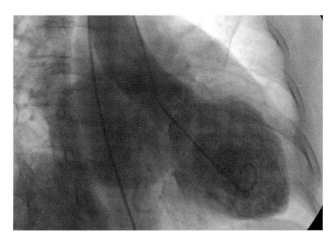

Figure 46.1 Left ventriculogram in an RAO (right anterior oblique) projection.

Cardiology Board Review: ECG, Hemodynamic and Angiographic Unknowns, First Edition. Edited by George A. Stouffer.
© 2019 John Wiley & Sons Ltd. Published 2019 by John Wiley & Sons Ltd.

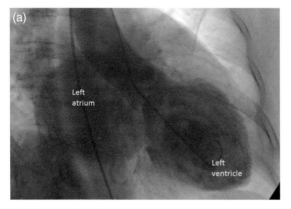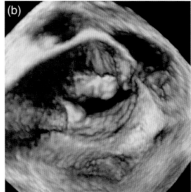

Figure 46.2 Left ventriculogram in an RAO projection with left atrium and left ventricle labeled (a) and 3D reconstruction of the mitral valve from TEE imaging (b)

Background

MR refers to backflow of blood from the left ventricle to the left atrium during systole due to incomplete closure of the mitral valve leaflets. This may be due to damage to the mitral valve leaflets, annulus, chordae tendinea, and/ or papillary muscles. It is the most common form of valvular heart disease with symptoms and hemodynamic significance ranging from trivial to severe. The Framingham Heart Study found MR of at least mild severity in 19% of men and women (Singh et al. 1999) and the Strong Heart Study found moderate to severe MR in 1.9% of men and 0.2% of women (Jones et al. 2001).

Etiology

MR can be categorized by etiology (primary versus secondary) or acuity (acute versus chronic). Primary MR results from disease or injury to the mitral valve leaflets, annulus, chordae tendineae, and/or papillary muscles, while secondary MR develops as a result of another cardiac pathology (usually left ventricular dilation).

The most common etiology of primary MR in developed countries is mitral valve prolapse (MVP) due to redundant mitral valve tissue and/or myxomatous degeneration of the mitral valve tissue. MVP is the largest cause of MR needing surgical repair in developed countries (Luxereau et al. 1991), however most patients with MVP do not require treatment. In the developing world, rheumatic heart disease remains a major cause of primary MR. Chronic rheumatic heart disease typically causes MR early in the disease process but may progress to mitral stenosis with or without MR in later adulthood (Marcus et al. 1994; Marijon et al. 2007). Endocarditis may also cause MR due to valvular tissue damage. Congenital defects of the mitral valve and connective tissue diseases (e.g. Marfan syndrome) are less common causes of MR.

Secondary MR is most commonly due to ischemic heart disease which may damage the papillary muscles or cause left ventricular dilation with consequent mitral annular dilation. Other cardiac pathologies that cause left ventricular dilation (dilated cardiomyopathy, aortic stenosis) may also cause secondary MR.

Pathogenesis

The regurgitant fraction of blood flows from the left ventricle into the left atrium, increasing left atrial pressure. This pressure can be communicated backwards to the pulmonary vasculature. In chronic MR, the cardiac chambers and pulmonary vasculature may compensate to manage these increased pressures: the left atrium will dilate and remodel (which may precipitate atrial fibrillation), the pulmonary vasculature will adapt, and the left ventricle will dilate and hypertrophy. These compensatory mechanisms may result in a prolonged asymptomatic phase in chronic MR. Over time the regurgitant fraction may increase, resulting in decreased cardiac output. In contrast to compensated chronic MR, acute MR due to papillary muscle or chordae tendineae rupture allows no time for compensation and left atrial and pulmonary vasculature pressures abruptly increase. Acute MR almost always presents with sudden onset of symptoms including severe shortness of breath (Yeung et al. 2018).

Clinical Presentation and Physical Exam

Presentation of MR depends on the acuity of the lesion, the severity of the regurgitation, and the degree of compensation. In cases of trivial, chronic, or well-compensated MR, patients may be asymptomatic for years. Acute or decompensated MR may present with signs of pulmonary edema (dyspnea, orthopnea, paroxysmal nocturnal dyspnea) or decreased forward perfusion (cool extremities, diaphoresis, hypotension, shock). Other common symptoms include fatigue, lower extremity edema, exercise intolerance, or palpitations.

The classic murmur of MR is a holosystolic murmur heard best at the apex that may radiate to the axilla, but murmur intensity does not correlate with MR severity and a murmur is not necessary for diagnosis. In severe MR, left ventricular enlargement may result in a leftward displacement of the apical impulse. Symptoms of acute MR may include a precordial thrill, S3, and pulmonary crackles.

Diagnosis and Management

Echocardiography is the most common modality for confirming MR and determining the etiology and severity of MR. Transthoracic echocardiography is the preferred screening and surveillance method while transesophageal echocardiography may give additional anatomic information prior to surgical repair. Cardiac MRI (magnetic resonance imaging) may detect mitral valve disease but has low spatial resolution and is used infrequently. Similarly, heart catheterization may show MR (as in the case study) but is rarely the first option for diagnosis when less invasive methods exist (Otto 2001).

Other studies may show nonspecific changes that can support the case of MR. Electrocardiography may show atrial fibrillation, left atrial enlargement (broad, notched P waves), or left ventricular enlargement and/or strain. Chest radiography may be normal or show cardiomegaly in chronic, severe MR (Otto 2001).

Treatment of MR depends on underlying etiology, symptoms, hemodynamic severity, and mitral valve anatomy. Primary MR is due to a structural problem of the mitral valve apparatus and surgical repair or replacement is the definitive treatment (Yeung et al. 2018). In eligible patients, repair of the native valve is preferred as it gives a durable result, preserves left ventricular function, eliminates the need for long term anticoagulation, and improves survival. However, some patients may be too ill or frail for surgery and less invasive methods, such as transcatheter mitral valve clip (e.g. MitraClip), may be an option. In cases of secondary MR, treatment should be aimed at the underlying primary etiology. Asymptomatic or hemodynamically insignificant MR should be monitored with serial echocardiograms (Nishimura et al. 2014).

References

Jones, E.C., Devereux, R.B., Roman, M.J. et al. (2001). Prevalence and correlates of mitral regurgitation in a population-based sample (the strong heart study). *The American Journal of Cardiology* 87 (3): 298–304.

Luxereau, P., Dorent, R., De Gevigney, G. et al. (1991). Aetiology of surgically treated mitral regurgitation. *European Heart Journal* 12: 2–4.

Marcus, R.H., Sareli, P., Pocock, W.A. et al. (1994). The spectrum of severe rheumatic mitral valve disease in a developing country. Correlations among clinical presentation, surgical pathologic findings, and hemodynamic sequelae. *Annals of Internal Medicine* 120 (3): 177–183.

Marijon, E., Ou, P., Celermajer, D.S. et al. (2007). Prevalence of rheumatic heart disease detected by echocardiographic screening. *The New England Journal of Medicine* 357 (5): 470–476. https://doi.org/10.1056/NEJMoa065085.

Nishimura, R.A., Otto, C.M., Bonow, R.O. et al. (2014). 2014 AHA/ACC guideline for the management of patients with valvular heart disease: a report of the American College of Cardiology/American Heart Association Task Force on Practice Guidelines. *Journal of the American College of Cardiology* 63 (22): e57–e185. https://doi.org/10.1016/j.jacc.2014.02.536.

Otto, C.M. (2001). Evaluation and management of chronic mitral regurgitation. *The New England Journal of Medicine* 345 (10): 740–746.

Singh, J.P., Evans, J.C., Levy, D. et al. (1999). Prevalence and clinical determinants of mitral, tricuspid, and aortic regurgitation (the Framingham heart study). *The American Journal of Cardiology* 83 (6): 897–902.

Yeung, M. and Griggs, T. (2018). Mitral valve disease. In: *Netter's Cardiology*, 3e (ed. G.A. Stouffer, M.S. Runge, C. Patterson and J.S. Rossi), 320–327. Elsevier.

Case 47: A 28-Year-Old Runner with Exercise-Induced Palpitations

You are asked to see a 28-year-old female who presented to the Emergency Department with complaints of palpitations. She was running on a treadmill at a local gym earlier this morning and noted that just before finishing she felt "tingly and like my heart rate was really high." The elevated heart rate persisted. At around noon she "got tingly and cold and started vomiting." She reports two similar episodes in the past. Approximately three months ago, similar symptoms occurred after she was running and lasted about three hours before spontaneously going away. The second episode was one month ago. She was running and noticed the symptoms after stopping. The episode lasted 45 minutes and resolved spontaneously. She has no past cardiac history and denies use of any caffeine, herbal medications, illicit drugs, or decongestants.

On physical examination, her blood pressure is 80/56 mmHg and heart rate is approximately 200 bpm. She is anxious and mildly diaphoretic but otherwise her exam is unremarkable. What does the ECG show and what clues does it provide in establishing a differential diagnosis (Figure 47.1)?

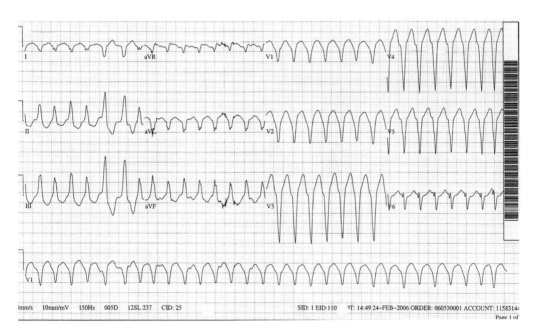

Figure 47.1 ECG on presentation.

Cardiology Board Review: ECG, Hemodynamic and Angiographic Unknowns, First Edition. Edited by George A. Stouffer.
© 2019 John Wiley & Sons Ltd. Published 2019 by John Wiley & Sons Ltd.

Additional Evaluation

The ECG shows a wide complex tachycardia. The patient was given adenosine, procainamide, and beta-blockers. Her rate accelerated to 220 bpm and she became hypotensive and lost consciousness. She was successfully defibrillated which resulted in the following ECG (Figure 47.2). What is the diagnosis?

Right Ventricular Outflow Tract Tachycardia

The ECG during the tachycardia shows a wide complex rhythm with a left bundle branch pattern (LBBB) and an inferior axis (QRS is positive in II, III, and aVF). The ECG following cardioversion is normal except for a rightward axis which can be a normal variant at this age. These ECG findings are consistent with a right ventricular outflow tract (RVOT) tachycardia. Also suggestive of this diagnosis is the fact that all episodes of palpitations occurred during or immediately after exercise.

RVOT tachycardia usually presents between the ages of 20 and 40 years old, with RVOT tachycardia being the most common type of ventricular tachycardia in patients under 40 years of age. There are various degrees of symptoms associated with RVOT tachycardia but in general two typical presentations have been described: nonsustained, repetitive, monomorphic ventricular tachycardia (VT) and paroxysmal, exercise-induced, sustained VT. The most common complaint is palpitations that are triggered by caffeine intake, stress, exercise (during or in recovery), or hormonal changes (in women).

In more than 80% of cases, the tachycardia originates from the RVOT leading to a LBBB configuration with an inferior axis. In most of these cases, the tachycardia originates from the muscular tissue just below the pulmonic valve. Recently, there have been several reports of the tachycardia originating from other sites such as within the pulmonary artery or the left ventricular outflow tract (LVOT). LVOT tachycardia is rare (<10% of outflow tract tachycardias) and may originate from either the supravalvular or infravalvular regions of the coronary cusps. LVOT tachycardia is suggested if the ECG during VT has an earlier precordial transition, more rightward axis, taller R waves in the inferior leads, and small R waves in lead V1.

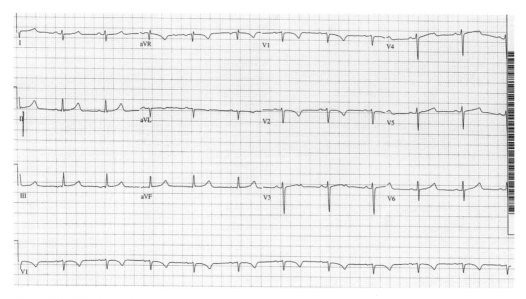

Figure 47.2 ECG after cardioversion.

Tachycardia in RVOT tachycardia is due to cAMP mediated triggered activity (triggered activity, rather than reentry or enhanced automaticity, is the cause of RVOT tachycardia). The tachycardia will generally terminate with adenosine administration but adenosine is not 100% effective as demonstrated by this case. In the electrophysiology laboratory, the tachycardia may be induced by programmed extrastimuli, by burst pacing the ventricle or atrium, or by infusion of isoproterenol. RVOT tachycardia can be treated with radiofrequency (RF) ablation with an overall success rate of >80%. In about 10% of cases, a second tachycardia with a different morphology will be present and may be a cause for recurrence despite successful ablation of the clinical ventricular tachycardia. A specific genetic defect has not been identified and the disease does not appear to be familial. Prognosis of patients with RVOT tachycardia is excellent and sudden death is rare.

The diagnosis of RVOT tachycardia is one of exclusion and thus a complete evaluation for the presence of structural heart disease must be undertaken including an evaluation for coronary ischemia, ventricular function, valvular heart disease, and congenital abnormalities. In particular, arrhythmogenic right ventricular dysplasia (ARVD) and sarcoidosis can mimic RVOT tachycardia. The ventricular tachycardia in ARVD may have LBBB with an inferior axis, similar to RVOT tachycardia (please see Chapter 11 for a more detailed discussion of ARVD).

There are various causes of VT in young adults in the absence of structural heart disease (generally defined as normal coronary angiography, right heart pressures, echocardiogram, and cardiac MRI [magnetic resonance imaging]). Brugada Syndrome and Long QT Syndrome can generally be identified by their characteristic ECG appearance when in normal sinus rhythm (please see Chapters 3, 25, 31, and 54 for more detailed discussion of these disorders). In the absence of structural heart disease and with a normal ECG during sinus rhythm, idiopathic left ventricular tachycardia (ILVT), idiopathic propranolol-sensitive VT (IPVT), catecholaminergic polymorphic VT (CPVT), and outflow tract tachycardias are in the differential diagnosis.

A starting point for the diagnosis of the cause of VT in the absence of structural heart disease is to examine the morphology of the tachycardia precipitating the clinical event. If the inciting clinical event is precipitated by polymorphic VT, torsades de pointes, or ventricular fibrillation, the differential diagnosis includes Long QT Syndrome, Brugada Syndrome, and CPVT. RVOT tachycardia, LVOT tachycardia, and ILVT cause monomorphic VT. The tachycardia associated with IPVT may be monomorphic or polymorphic. Most cases of ILVT are verapamil-sensitive intrafascicular tachycardias with a right bundle branch block (RBBB) and left-axis configuration in 90–95% of cases (the rest have RBBB with a right-axis pattern). CPVT is characterized by a uniform pattern of bidirectional polymorphic VT that can be easily and reproducibly induced during exercise, emotional stress, or catecholamine infusion.

This patient had no evidence of structural heart disease after an extensive evaluation. She underwent successful catheter ablation of a focus in the RVOT and resumed her running.

Further Reading

Joshi, S. and Wilber, D.J. (2005). Ablation of idiopathic right ventricular outflow tract tachycardia: current perspectives. *Journal of Cardiovascular Electrophysiology* 16: S52–S58.

Saeid, A.K., Klein, G.J., and Leong-Sit, P. (2016). Sustained ventricular tachycardia in apparently normal hearts: medical therapy should be the first step in management. *Cardiac Electrophysiology Clinics* 8 (3): 631–639.

Case 48: A 43-Year-Old Man with Chest Pain and an Episode of Syncope

A 43-year-old male with a past medical history of treated hypertension arrives at the Emergency Department (ED) via private vehicle with complaints of a fainting episode followed by the development of substernal chest pressure. Ninety minutes prior to arrival at the ED he was walking from the kitchen to the couch and passed out for a few seconds (per his wife), hitting his head on the way down. Upon waking he "felt fine" but his wife called EMS (Emergency Medical Services) who evaluated him and determined that he was dehydrated and left. Thirty minutes later he had severe substernal chest

pressure which has persisted. What clues does the ECG provide in establishing a differential diagnosis (Figure 48.1)?

Inferior-Posterior Myocardial Infarction

Myocardial infarction (MI) can be readily diagnosed on this ECG. There is ST elevation in leads II, III, and AVF, consistent with an injury pattern involving the inferior wall. There is ST depression in V2–V4 which probably represents posterior wall

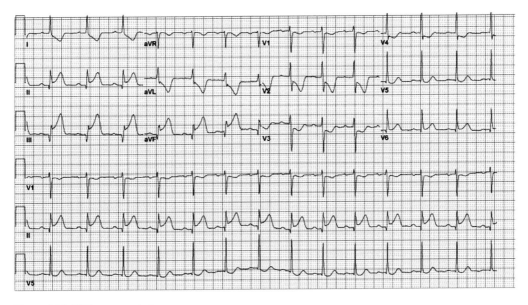

Figure 48.1 ECG on presentation.

Cardiology Board Review: ECG, Hemodynamic and Angiographic Unknowns, First Edition. Edited by George A. Stouffer.
© 2019 John Wiley & Sons Ltd. Published 2019 by John Wiley & Sons Ltd.

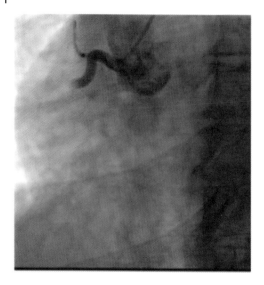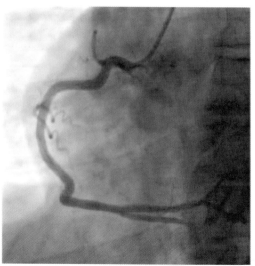

Figure 48.2 Angiograms in an LAO (left anterior oblique) projection before and after percutaneous coronary intervention.

infarction (anterior ST depression is equivalent to posterior ST elevation). There is also ST depression in I and aVL. Taken together, these changes are consistent with a large MI involving the inferior, posterior, and lateral walls. Emergent angiography showed proximal occlusion of a large right coronary artery (Figure 48.2).

Localizing coronary ischemia based on ECG findings is not an exact science but some generalities are useful. Based on typical anatomy, the left anterior descending (LAD) coronary artery and branches usually supply the anterior and anterolateral walls of the left ventricle and the anterior two-thirds of the septum. The left circumflex coronary artery and branches usually supply the posterolateral wall of the left ventricle. The right coronary artery supplies the right ventricle, the inferior and true posterior walls of the left ventricle, and the posterior third of the septum. In 15–30% of individuals, the posterior descending coronary artery (which supplies the inferior wall) will originate from the left circumflex. Rarely, the LAD will extend around the apex and onto the inferior wall.

Inferior wall infarcts are characterized by changes in the inferior leads – II, III, and aVF (Table 48.1). An anterior wall infarct involves

Table 48.1 Localization of myocardial infarction (MI) based on ECG changes according to the American Heart Association.

Leads	Portion of heart involved
II, III, aVf	Inferior wall
V1, V2	Septum
V1 – V3 (sometimes V4)	Anteroseptal
V3, V4 (sometimes V2)	Anterior wall
V3, V4	Apical
I, aVL, V5, V6	Lateral wall
V1 – V6	Extensive anterior wall
V1 – V3 (ST depression)	Posterior wall

leads V3 and V4. If leads V1 and V2 are also involved it is sometimes labeled an anteroseptal infarct, and if leads V5 and V6 ± leads I and aVL are involved it is labeled an anterolateral infarct. ST elevation in leads V1–V6 is characteristic of an extensive anterior wall MI. Lateral wall infarcts are reflected in leads I and aVL ± V5 and V6. The "posterior wall" has no direct facing leads, however infarction of this territory can be reflected by a large R wave in V1 or ST depression in leads V1–V4. The use of the term "posterior wall" to identify the basal part of the left ventricle that lies on the diaphragm has fallen out of favor among some cardiologists who believe it is anatomically inaccurate and thus this terminology may change in the future. In a recent AHA/ACC/HRS (American Heart Association/American College of Cardiology/Heart Rhythm Society) Scientific Statement however, the consensus was that there was insufficient evidence to change the existing terminology and they recommended using the following classifications: anterior, inferior, posterior, lateral, extensive anterior, and right ventricular MI and MI in the presence of bundle branch block.

The ECG is a tremendously useful tool in patients with chest pain and it is the most important variable in determining whether patients receive emergent reperfusion therapy. It is important however to emphasize that the specificity of the ECG in localizing MI is limited by: (i) individual variations in coronary anatomy; (ii) presence of coronary artery disease in the non-infarct related artery; (iii) previous MI; and (iv) inadequate representation of the posterior, lateral, and apical walls of the left ventricle. The use of ECGs with more than 12 channels that better reflect the lateral and posterior walls are under investigation.

Right ventricular infarction occurs in a significant percentage of patients with inferior MI. To diagnose this condition based on ECG findings, the precordial leads should be placed on the right side of the chest in a mirror image of usual placement (Figure 48.3). The most sensitive ECG sign of right ventricular infarction is ST segment elevation of more than 1 mm in lead V_4R with an upright T wave in that lead. Other ECG findings suggestive of RV infarction include ST elevation in leads V3R, V5R, V6R, or V_1 in association with ST segment elevation in leads II, III, and aVF.

During ischemic events, ECG changes evolve over time. These changes are variable depending on reperfusion, the size and location of the MI, and other factors. An initial finding after the onset of ischemia may be

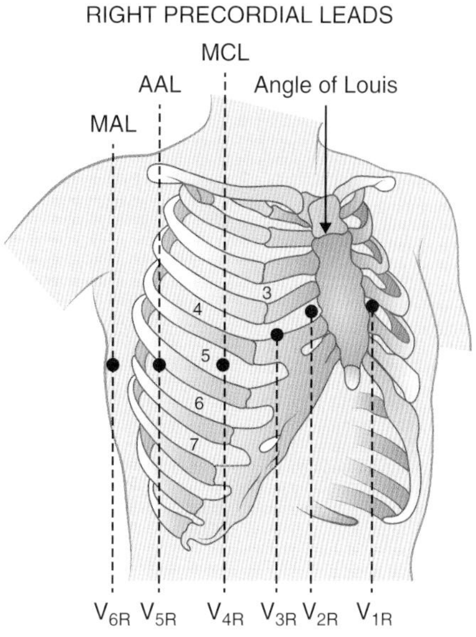

Figure 48.3 Right-sided ECG leads used in the diagnosis of right ventricular infarction.

"hyperacute" T wave changes – the appearance of tall T waves in leads corresponding to a vascular bed supplied by a coronary artery. This is followed by ST elevation. ST elevation will resolve over time with re-establishment of blood supply (either via reperfusion or development of collaterals). ST segment resolution is associated with T wave inversion and occasionally with Q wave formation (depending on the extent of the infarct). A pathological Q wave is defined as an initial downward deflection that persists for 40 ms or more in any lead except III and aVR. An ECG on this patient, taken 36 hours after the event, shows resolution of ST elevation, development of Q waves, and T wave inversion (Figure 48.4). Over time, the T wave will return to an upright position in most individuals. Persistent ST elevation, especially in the setting of Q waves, is a marker of aneurysm formation.

Several studies have looked at ECG findings that help identify which artery is involved in an inferior wall MI. The major findings of these studies are that: (i) ST segment elevation in lead III > lead II; (ii) ST segment depression of more than 1 mm in leads I and aVL; or (iii) ST segment elevation in lead V_1

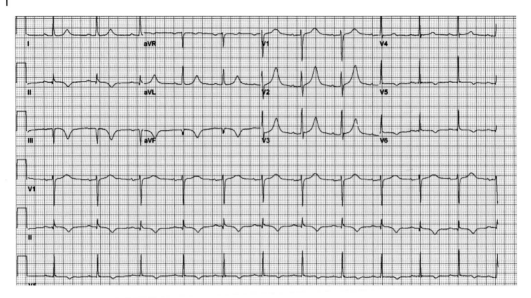

Figure 48.4 ECG taken 36 hours after initial presentation.

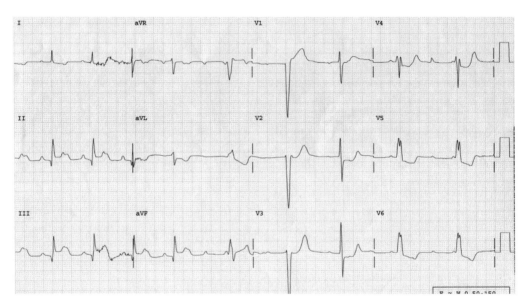

Figure 48.5 Inferior myocardial infarction (MI) with second and third degree atrioventricular (AV) block.

suggest right coronary artery involvement. An ST segment vector directed toward the left (i.e. lead II > lead III) suggests circumflex involvement.

Arrhythmias, including atrioventricular (AV) block, accelerated idioventricular rhythm, or ventricular arrhythmias are common during inferior MI. An ECG with second and third degree AV block in the setting of an inferior MI from a different patient is shown in Figure 48.5. AV block generally occurs early (within a few hours) in an inferior MI as a result of heightened vagal tone. Complete AV block is generally associated with a narrow complex escape rhythm of between 40 and 60 beats per minute.

Further Reading

Levine, G.N., Bates, E.R., Blankenship, J.C. et al. (2016). 2015 ACC/AHA/SCAI Focused Update on Primary Percutaneous Coronary Intervention for Patients With ST-Elevation Myocardial Infarction. *Journal of the American College of Cardiology* 67: 1235–1250. https://doi.org/10.1016/j.jacc.2015.10.005.

Thygesen, K., Alpert, J.S., Jaffe, A.S. et al. (2018). Fourth universal definition of myocardial infarction. *Journal of the American College of Cardiology* 72 (18): 2231–2264.

Wagner, G.S., Macfarlane, P., Wellens, H. et al. (2009). AHA/ACCF/HRS recommendations for the standardization and interpretation of the electrocardiogram: part VI: acute ischemia/infarction a scientific statement from the American Heart Association Electrocardiography and Arrhythmias Committee, Council on Clinical Cardiology; the American College of Cardiology Foundation; and the Heart Rhythm Society endorsed by the International Society for Computerized Electrocardiology. *Journal of the American College of Cardiology* 53 (11): 1003–1011.

Case 49: A 50-Year-Old Man with Worsening Cough and Dyspnea

A 50-year-old male is referred to you for follow-up care after being recently hospitalized. He had no significant past medical history before presenting to the Emergency Department two weeks ago with a three-day history of cough productive of rusty-colored sputum and shortness of breath. Chest x-ray showed bilateral infiltrates with small bilateral pleural effusions. The patient was treated with ceftriaxone and azithromycin with some symptomatic improvement. His main complaint at this point is persistent dyspnea on exertion. On your exam, you hear a soft diastolic murmur that was not appreciated in the Emergency Department. You obtain an ECG which is shown below.

What does the ECG show (Figure 49.1)?

Mitral Stenosis

The ECG shows evidence of left atrial (LA) enlargement, right axis deviation, right ventricular hypertrophy (RVH), and P–mitrale (lead II). Of the valvular diseases, only a few can be diagnosed from the ECG. Mitral stenosis (MS) is one of these and is strongly suggested, in the appropriate patient population,

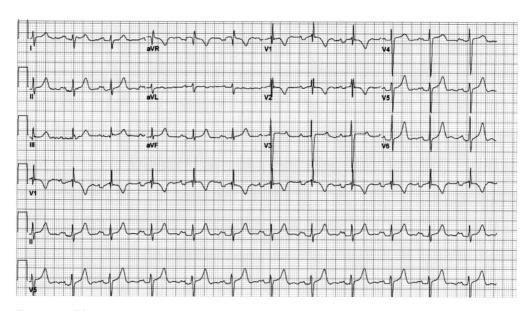

Figure 49.1 ECG on presentation.

Cardiology Board Review: ECG, Hemodynamic and Angiographic Unknowns, First Edition. Edited by George A. Stouffer.
© 2019 John Wiley & Sons Ltd. Published 2019 by John Wiley & Sons Ltd.

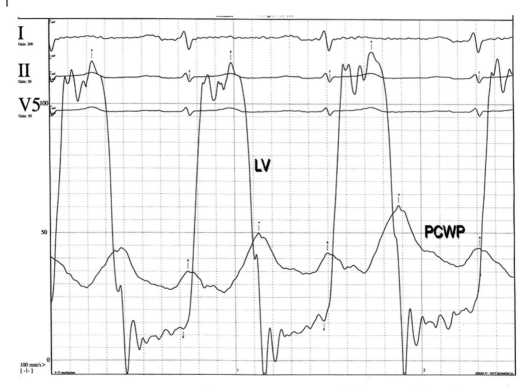

Figure 49.2 Simultaneous recording of left ventricular pressure (LV) and pulmonary capillary wedge pressure (PCWP).

by the presence of LA enlargement and RVH in the absence of left ventricular dysfunction. The diastolic murmur heard on examination is consistent with the diagnosis of MS.

Echocardiography was performed followed by left and right heart catheterization.

This pressure tracing (Figure 49.2) confirms the diagnosis of severe MS with a mean transmitral diastolic pressure gradient of 25 mmHg. The calculated mitral valve area was 0.7 cm^2. The patient had pulmonary hypertension with pulmonary artery pressures of 68/30 mmHg.

The cross-sectional area of the mitral valve is 4–6 cm^2 in healthy adults. MS occurs when this area decreases, resulting in increased resistance to flow from the LA to left ventricle (LV) and increased LA pressure. The increased LA pressure is transmitted to the pulmonary circulation, resulting in elevated right heart pressures. MS is a progressive disorder with symptoms worsening as mitral

valve area decreases. Symptoms do not usually appear until mitral valve area <2 cm^2. Initially symptoms occur only with exertion, emotional stress, or pregnancy and consist primarily of dyspnea. Symptoms can progress over time as the valve opening declines further and in severe cases will eventually include dyspnea at rest, orthopnea, and paroxysmal nocturnal dyspnea. More rarely, there may be angina, palpitations, recumbent cough, and/or hemoptysis.

The severity of MS can be assessed by echocardiography or cardiac catheterization. At cardiac catheterization, the mitral valve gradient may be directly measured by comparing simultaneous pressures in the LV and LA (either by directly measuring LA pressures or using pulmonary capillary wedge pressure [PCWP]). The gradient across the mitral valve should be measured using an average of five cardiac cycles in patients with normal sinus rhythm and 10 cardiac cycles in patients with atrial fibrillation. In order to avoid a transseptal puncture, PCWP is commonly used in place of LA pressure. In this scenario, it is essential to ensure that an accurate wedge tracing is obtained.

The severity of obstruction in MS can be quantified using mitral valve area or mean gradient. Mitral valve area remains the standard used in most laboratories because it includes the three major hemodynamic variables: transvalvular pressure gradient, cardiac output, and diastolic filling period. By convention, a mitral valve area $<1\,cm^2$ is considered severe MS; a valve area of $1–1.5\,cm^2$ is moderate stenosis and a valve area $1.5–2\,cm^2$ is mild stenosis. By convention, mean gradient $>10\,mmHg$, $5–10\,mmHg$, and $<5\,mmHg$ at rest are severe, moderate, and mild MS, respectively. Transvalvular gradient will increase in direct proportion to flow across the valve and thus conditions that increase cardiac output (e.g. anemia, hyperthyroidism, anxiety, exercise, mitral regurgitation) will result in increased gradients.

Almost all cases of MS are rheumatic in origin. Isolated MS occurs in 40% of all patients presenting with rheumatic heart disease and women with MS outnumber men by approximately 2:1. Rheumatic mitral valve changes including thickening of the mitral valve leaflets, calcification, and commissural fusion occur over the course of decades. Other rare causes of MS include systemic lupus erythematosis, rheumatoid arthritis, carcinoid, mucopolysaccharidosis, mitral annular calcification, and congenital valve deformity. Conditions that cause increased LA pressure can mimic MS. Examples include LA myxoma, pulmonary vein obstruction, and cor triatriatum (a thin membrane across the left atrium which obstructs pulmonary venous inflow).

Further Reading

Carabello, B.A. (2005). Modern management of mitral stenosis. *Circulation* 112: 432–437.

Lung, B. and Vahanian, A. (2011). Epidemiology of valvular heart disease in the adult. *Nature Reviews Cardiology* 8 (3): 162–172.

Nishimura, R.A., Otto, C.M., Bonow, R.O. et al. (2014). 2014 AHA/ACC guideline for the management of patients with valvular heart disease: a report of the American College of Cardiology/American Heart Association Task Force on Practice Guidelines. *Journal of the American College of Cardiology* 63 (22): e57–e185.

Nishimura, R.A., Otto, C.M., Bonow, R.O. et al. (2017). 2017 AHA/ACC focused update of the 2014 AHA/ACC guideline for the management of patients with valvular heart disease: a report of the American College of Cardiology/American Heart Association Task Force on Clinical Practice Guidelines. *Journal of the American College of Cardiology* 70 (2): 252–289.

Case 50: Unsuspected Congenital Heart Disease in a 26-Year-Old Woman

A 26-year-old female is arrested and incarcerated. While in custody, she complains of shortness of breath. She is brought to the Emergency Department (ED) where an ECG is done. The ED physician asks you to see the patient and comment on the ECG.

On your physical examination, cyanosis is apparent. Vital signs includes a blood pressure of 125/75 mmHg, a heart rate of 74 bpm, and oxygen saturation of 78% on room air.

You ask her if her shortness of breath has ever been evaluated and she reports that she

has not seen a physician in over 10 years. What are the important findings from this ECG (Figure 50.1)?

Discussion

This ECG is distinctly abnormal for a 26-year-old female. It shows right axis deviation, right ventricular hypertrophy (RVH), and right atrial (RA) enlargement. The diffuse ST and T wave abnormalities (especially those in the

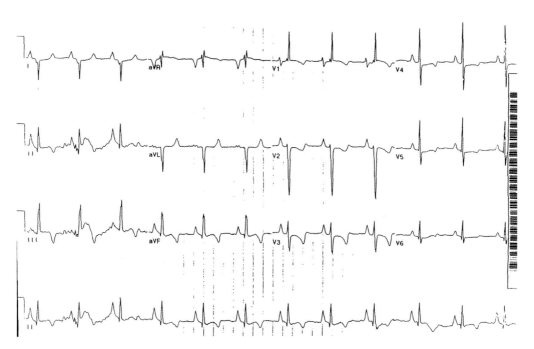

Figure 50.1 ECG on presentation.

Cardiology Board Review: ECG, Hemodynamic and Angiographic Unknowns, First Edition. Edited by George A. Stouffer.
© 2019 John Wiley & Sons Ltd. Published 2019 by John Wiley & Sons Ltd.

right precordial leads) are most likely due to right ventricular "strain" (i.e. RVH with strain). These findings are all highly suggestive of increased RV (right ventricular) and RA pressures. The differential diagnosis in a patient of this age would include disorders causing pulmonary hypertension (e.g. mitral stenosis, primary pulmonary hypertension, an atrial septal defect with pulmonary hypertension), and disorders causing RV pressure or volume overload (e.g. pulmonic stenosis, ventricular septal defect). The next step in evaluation of this patient would be an echocardiogram which was done and had findings consistent with tetralogy of Fallot.

The patient had been diagnosed at birth and her family was told that she would need surgery but she had not sought medical care until she was incarcerated. The natural history of tetralogy of Fallot, if uncorrected, is progressive right heart failure and hypoxemia and it is unusual for a patient to survive for 26 years. During her hospitalization, this patient's O$_2$ saturation while breathing room air was in the 60s and 70s.

Tetralogy of Fallot is characterized by a large ventricular septal defect, an "overriding" aorta, RV outflow tract obstruction (that is generally subvalvular but may also be valvular, supravalvular, or in the pulmonary arterial branches), and RVH. Most adults with uncorrected tetralogy of Fallot have substantial right-to-left shunting and it is the most common cyanotic congenital heart defect after infancy. The rate of survival without surgery is dismal with only 3% alive at 40 years. ECGs in adults with uncorrected tetralogy of Fallot are almost always abnormal, with the most common abnormalities being RA enlargement, right axis deviation, and RVH.

Further Reading

Downing, T.E. and Kim, Y.Y. (2015). Tetralogy of Fallot: general principles of management. *Cardiology clinics* 33 (4): 531–541.

Stout, K.K., Daniels, C.J., Aboulhosn, J.A. et al. (2018 Aug 10). 2018 AHA/ACC Guideline for the management of Adults With Congenital Heart Disease: A Report of the American College of Cardiology/American Heart Association Task Force on Clinical Practice Guidelines. *Journal of the American College of Cardiology* 73: 1494–1563. https://doi.org/10.1016/j.jacc.2018.08.1028.

Case 51: How Likely Is This Patient to Have a Bad Outcome?

Risk Stratification in Non-ST Elevation Myocardial Infarction (NSTEMI)

A 68-year-old male with hypertension, hyperlipidemia, and diabetes mellitus presents to the Emergency Department with two episodes of acute chest pain at rest. He describes his chest pain as substernal pressure, radiating to his jaw, associated with nausea and diaphoresis, worse with exertion, and lasting for 30 minutes. His first episode of chest pain occurred this morning. His second episode of chest pain occurred several hours later, prompting him to go to the emergency room. His current medications are aspirin 81 mg daily, atorvastatin 20 mg daily, lisinopril 10 mg daily, metformin 500 mg twice a day, and insulin. He has smoked one pack of cigarettes per day for 30 years. His family history is notable for his father having a myocardial infarction (MI) at age 50.

His vital signs include a blood pressure of 136/88 mmHg, a pulse of 78 bpm, a respiratory rate of 16, and an oxygen saturation of 98% on room air. Cardiovascular examination demonstrates a regular rate and rhythm, with no murmurs, rubs, or gallops. His lungs are clear on auscultation. He has no evidence of jugular venous distension. Extremities are warm with palpable pulses and no edema.

A 12-lead electrocardiogram (ECG) is shown below (Figure 51.1). Laboratory values are notable for a troponin I of 1.25 ng/ml.

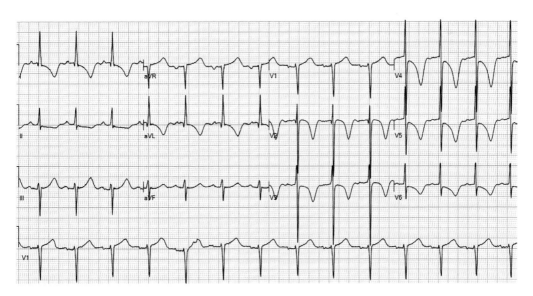

Figure 51.1 ECG on presentation.

Cardiology Board Review: ECG, Hemodynamic and Angiographic Unknowns, First Edition. Edited by George A. Stouffer.
© 2019 John Wiley & Sons Ltd. Published 2019 by John Wiley & Sons Ltd.

Basic metabolic panel, complete blood count, and thyroid stimulating hormone are normal. He is given aspirin 325 mg, clopidogrel 300 mg, and a bolus of heparin; started on a continuous heparin infusion; and admitted to the cardiology service. He is currently free of chest pain.

What is his Thrombolysis in Myocardial Infarction (TIMI) risk score and what is the next best step in his management?

Discussion

The patient presents with ischemic symptoms, evidence of anterior and lateral ST segment depressions with deep T wave inversions on ECG, and elevated cardiac troponin; consistent with a non-ST elevation myocardial infarction (NSTEMI). He received antiplatelet and antithrombin therapies which are both class 1 recommendations. In the TIMI NSTEMI risk score, each of the following is given one point: (i) age greater than 65 years; (ii) three of more risk factors for coronary artery disease (CAD); (iii) aspirin use in the past seven days; (iv) two or more episodes of angina in the past 24 hours; (v) ST segment changes ≥0.5 mm on ECG; (vi) elevated cardiac biomarker levels; and (vii) significant coronary artery stenosis. He has a TIMI score of 6 which corresponds to a 41% risk of 14-day all-cause mortality, new or recurrent MI, or severe recurrent ischemia requiring urgent revascularization (risk with scores of 0–6 are 5, 5, 8, 13, 20, 26, and 41%, respectively). The next best step in his management is to refer him for invasive coronary angiography to define his coronary anatomy, and then to perform either percutaneous or surgical revascularization as needed.

Figure 51.2 shows a left coronary angiogram after the administration of nitroglycerin.

The patient has angiographic evidence of a 90% stenosis in the left anterior descending (LAD) coronary artery which is the culprit lesion for his NSTEMI.

Acute coronary syndromes (ACS) define the spectrum of conditions during which an

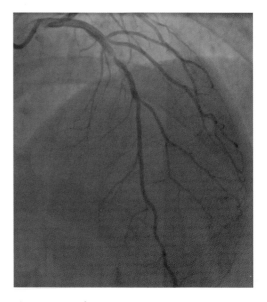

Figure 51.2 Left coronary angiography in an AP (anteroposterior) cranial view.

abrupt reduction in coronary blood flow leads to acute myocardial ischemia or MI (Arbab-Zadeh et al. 2012; Thygesen et al. 2018; Libby 2013; Amsterdam et al. 2014). These conditions are classified based on electrocardiographic findings and cardiac troponin levels that reflect the underlying pathology. An ST elevation myocardial infarction (STEMI) is defined as ECG evidence of ST segment elevation in at least two contiguous leads in a patient with characteristic symptoms and occurs when an acute thrombotic occlusion of a coronary artery leads to transmural infarction. A NSTEMI is defined as increased troponin levels in the absence of ST segment elevation on ECG, and occurs when an acute thrombotic event in a coronary artery leads to a nontransmural infarction (usually due to embolization of thrombus from the site of the ruptured plaque into the distal vasculature). Unstable angina (UA) is not associated with increased troponin levels but can be associated with transient ECG changes and reflects an acute flow-limiting plaque that leads to transient ischemia without infarction. Patients with NSTEMI and UA are grouped into the same clinical population, with respect to prognostication and management.

The primary pathophysiology of ACS in a type 1 MI (there are five types of MI but type 1 is the most common) is a spontaneous atherosclerotic plaque rupture or erosion that results in intraluminal thrombosis in one or more coronary arteries, leading to prolonged myocardial ischemia and ultimately myocardial cell death (Thygesen et al. 2018). The culprit plaque is typically composed of a large necrotic lipid-rich core, covered by a thin fibrous cap (Arbab-Zadeh et al. 2012; Thygesen et al. 2018; Libby 2013). A complex interplay of factors involving coronary blood flow dynamics, plaque characteristics, inflammatory conditions, metabolic conditions, environmental conditions, and neurohormonal imbalance is thought to cause plaque rupture (Arbab-Zadeh et al. 2012). In the setting of plaque rupture, tissue factor is released from macrophages in the necrotic core and comes into contact with blood in the coronary artery, activating the coagulation cascade with subsequent generation of thrombin and leading to platelet activation and aggregation (Libby 2013). This culminates in acute coronary thrombosis resulting in myocardial ischemia and infarction.

Diagnostic Evaluation

A comprehensive history and physical exam are essential in the initial evaluation of patients with suspected NSTEMI/UA (Amsterdam et al. 2014). Patients typically present with angina which is described as substernal pain or pressure, occurring with exertion or at rest, worse with exertion and/or emotional stress, improving with rest and/or nitroglycerin, and lasting for at least 10–15 minutes. The pain may radiate to the shoulders, arms, neck, or jaw. There may be associated symptoms such as dyspnea, diaphoresis, nausea, dizziness, and syncope. Patients can have atypical presentations and this is more common in those who are at least 75 years old, are female, have diabetes

mellitus, or have impaired renal function. These patients can present with angina-equivalent symptoms of dyspnea, diaphoresis, nausea, fatigue, and/or syncope instead of chest pain or pressure. While a history of known CAD, percutaneous coronary intervention (PCI), or coronary artery bypass graft (CABG) surgery increases the likelihood of ACS; the traditional risk factors for atherosclerotic cardiovascular disease including age, male sex, family history of premature coronary artery disease, hypertension, hyperlipidemia, smoking, diabetes mellitus, and renal insufficiency also increase the pretest probability of NSTEMI/UA.

Physical exam can be normal but may identify the presence of the following complications of MI: ischemic heart failure (third heart sound, pulmonary rales, jugular venous distension, hepatojugular reflex, peripheral edema), cardiogenic shock (profound hypotension with tachycardia, cool extremities, signs of heart failure), mitral regurgitation due to papillary muscle ischemia or infarction (apical holosystolic murmur with pulmonary rales), or ischemic conduction disease (profound bradycardia).

Patients with chest pain or angina-equivalent symptoms should have a 12-lead ECG performed within the first 10 minutes followed by serial ECGs if the initial ECG is not diagnostic or if there are new or recurrent symptoms (Amsterdam et al. 2014). Concerning ECG findings in NSTEMI/UA include ST segment depressions in at least two contiguous leads, new T-wave inversions in at least two contiguous leads, a new left or right bundle branch block, a new high-degree AV block, and ventricular ectopy such as premature ventricular contractions or ventricular tachycardia.

Patients with chest pain or angina-equivalent symptoms should also have a cardiac troponin level measured at initial presentation and again at three to six hours after symptom onset (Amsterdam et al. 2014). A troponin value that is above the 99th percentile of the upper reference level and a repeat troponin value that reflects a serial increase or decrease by at least 20% are considered diagnostic for acute MI (Keller et al. 2011; Newby et al. 2012; Thygesen et al. 2018; Amsterdam et al. 2014). In addition, the magnitude of troponin elevation can be useful for the prognostication of infarct size (Giannitsis et al. 2008). Other cardiac biomarker assays including creatine kinase (CK-MB) and myoglobin should not be used for the diagnosis of acute MI (Amsterdam et al. 2014).

Risk Stratification

Given the increased risk of morbidity and mortality, patients with ACS should undergo early diagnosis and risk stratification (Amsterdam et al. 2014). There are two widely used risk prediction models in patients with NSTEMI/UA. The TIMI risk model has been validated in multiple studies and uses seven indicators to generate a score: age greater than 65 years; at least three CAD risk factors (hypertension, hyperlipidemia, diabetes mellitus, smoking, family history); known CAD with a major coronary artery stenosis of at least 50%; recent aspirin use in the past seven days; severe angina with at least two episodes in the past 24 hours; ECG findings of ST segment changes; and elevated cardiac biomarkers (Antman et al. 2000; Than et al. 2012). Each indicator adds one point to the total score which ultimately corresponds to a calculated risk of 14-day all-cause mortality, new or recurrent MI, or severe recurrent ischemia requiring urgent revascularization. The Global Registry of Acute Coronary Events (GRACE) risk model has also been validated and incorporates numerous indicators (age, vitals, ECG findings of ST segment changes, elevated cardiac biomarkers, serum creatinine, and Killip class for heart failure) to generate a score that is associated with a calculated risk of in-hospital and six-month mortality (Granger et al. 2003; Eagle et al. 2004; Abu-Assi et al. 2010).

Management

All patients with NSTEMI/UA should be stabilized on initial presentation and then started on evidence-based medical therapies in a timely manner. These therapies include dual anti-platelet therapy (DAPT), anticoagulation, nitrates, beta-blockers, angiotensin-converting enzyme (ACE) inhibitors or angiotensin receptor blockers (ARB), and high-intensity statins.

Antithrombotic therapies are the cornerstone of medical therapy in ACS. Patients with NSTEMI/UA should be on DAPT with aspirin and a P2Y12 inhibitor for at least 12 months (Amsterdam et al. 2014; Levine et al. 2016). Nonenteric-coated aspirin should be given as soon as possible (at a loading dose of 162–325 mg) and should be continued indefinitely. Patients who do not undergo PCI can receive either clopidogrel (with a loading dose of 300 or 600 mg followed by a maintenance dose of 75 mg daily) or ticagrelor (with a loading dose of 180 mg followed by a maintenance dose of 90 mg twice daily) (Mehta et al. 2001; Wallentin et al. 2009; Amsterdam et al. 2014; Levine et al. 2016). Following PCI, patients can receive clopidogrel, ticagrelor, or prasugrel (with a loading dose of 60 mg and a maintenance dose of 10 mg daily) (Mehta et al. 2001; Wiviott et al. 2007; Wallentin et al. 2009; Amsterdam et al. 2014; Levine et al. 2016). Recent studies have demonstrated that patients with a CYP2C19 loss-of-function allele who take clopidogrel following PCI have an increased risk of adverse cardiovascular events and that a CYP2C19 genotype-guided DAPT strategy is feasible (Cavallari et al. 2018; Lee et al. 2018). Finally, anticoagulation is administered as soon as possible in one of the following formulations: intravenous unfractionated heparin for 48 hours or until PCI is performed, intravenous bivalirudin until PCI is performed in patients who undergo an early invasive strategy, subcutaneous enoxaparin or fondaparinux for the duration of the hospitalization or until PCI is performed.

Antianginal therapy with sublingual nitroglycerin should be administered every five minutes as needed for a total of three doses. Patients who have persistent ischemia, uncontrolled hypertension, or decompensated heart failure can be started on intravenous nitroglycerin. Oral beta-blocker therapy is recommended within the first 24 hours in patients who do not have decompensated heart failure or low cardiac output, an increased risk of cardiogenic shock, or a contraindication to beta blockade (Chen et al. 2005; Amsterdam et al. 2014). Oral nondihydropyridine calcium channel blocker therapy (verapamil or diltiazem) can be given to patients when beta-blocker therapy is contraindicated, not successful, or cause unacceptable side effects (Amsterdam et al. 2014). ACE inhibitors are recommended in patients with a left ventricular ejection fraction less than 40% and in those with hypertension, diabetes mellitus, or stable chronic kidney disease; those who are not tolerant to ACE inhibitors can receive ARB (GISSI-3 Group 1994; Amsterdam et al. 2014). Finally, high-intensity statin therapy is recommended in all patients with NSTEMI/UA (Cannon et al. 2004; Amsterdam et al. 2014).

Based on their risk profile and clinical presentation, patients with NSTEMI/UA can be managed with an early invasive strategy or ischemia-guided strategy (Boden et al. 1998; Cannon et al. 2001; Fox et al. 2002; de Winter et al. 2005; Damman et al. 2010; Amsterdam et al. 2014). An early invasive strategy is defined as proceeding with invasive coronary angiography with the intent to perform percutaneous or surgical revascularization based on coronary anatomy, and is recommend in high-risk patients including those with an elevated TIMI score (at least 2), an elevated GRACE score (at least 109), troponin elevation, new ECG changes, newly reduced left ventricular systolic function, history of diabetes mellitus or renal insufficiency, prior PCI in the past six months, or prior CABG surgery. Patients with hemodynamic instability, electrical instability (sustained ventricular tachycardia or ventricular fibrillation), recurrent ischemia despite intensive medical therapy, or new or worsening heart failure or mitral regurgitation should undergo an immediate or urgent invasive strategy. On the other hand, low-risk patients, including those with a low TIMI score (less than 2), a low GRACE score (less than 109), no troponin elevations, and no ECG changes can be candidates for an ischemia-guided strategy. Using this strategy, referral for invasive coronary angiography occurs only with recurrent symptoms or if there is objective evidence of ischemia on non-invasive stress testing.

Finally, following the initiation of evidence-based medical therapies and provision of coronary revascularization if needed, patients with NSTEMI/UA should undergo risk factor modification and secondary prevention strategies. These strategies include smoking cessation, nutrition and physical activity counseling, referral to cardiac rehabilitation, optimization of comorbidities (specifically hypertension, hyperlipidemia, diabetes mellitus, obesity, and heart failure), and timely post-discharge follow-up with care coordination. While survival rates following acute MI have improved in the contemporary era of cardiology, reduction in hospital readmissions and comorbidities following acute ischemic heart disease remain a target for investigation and quality improvement.

References

Abu-Assi, E., Ferreira-Gonzalez, I., Ribera, A. et al. (2010). Do GRACE (Global Registry of Acute Coronary Events) risk scores still maintain their performance for predicting mortality in the era of contemporary management of acute coronary syndromes? *American Heart Journal* 160 (5): 826–834.

Amsterdam, E.A., Wenger, N.K., Brindis, R.G. et al. (2014). 2014 AHA/ACC guideline for the management of patients with non-ST-elevation acute coronary syndromes: a report of the American College of Cardiology/American Heart Association Task Force on Practice Guidelines. *Journal of the American College of Cardiology* 64 (24): e139–e228.

Antman, E.M., Cohen, M., Bernink, P.J. et al. (2000). The TIMI risk score for unstable angina/non-ST elevation MI: a method for prognostication and therapeutic decision making. *Journal of the American Medical Association* 284 (7): 835–842.

Arbab-Zadeh, A., Nakano, M., Virmani, R. et al. (2012). Acute coronary events. *Circulation* 125 (9): 1147–1156.

Boden, W.E., O'Rourke, R.A., Crawford, M.H. et al. (1998). Outcomes in patients with acute non-Q-wave myocardial infarction randomly assigned to an invasive as compared with a conservative management strategy. *The New England Journal of Medicine* 338 (25): 1785–1792.

Cannon, C.P., Braunwald, E., McCabe, C.H. et al. (2004). Intensive versus moderate lipid lowering with statins after acute coronary syndromes. *The New England Journal of Medicine* 350 (15): 1495–1504.

Cannon, C.P., Weintraub, W.S., Demopoulos, L.A. et al. (2001). Comparison of early invasive and conservative strategies in patients with unstable coronary syndromes treated with the glycoprotein IIb/IIIa inhibitor tirofiban. *The New England Journal of Medicine* 344 (25): 1879–1887.

Cavallari, L.H., Lee, C.R., Beitelshees, A.L. et al. (2018). Multisite investigation of outcomes with implementation of CYP2C19 genotype-guided antiplatelet therapy after percutaneous coronary intervention. *JACC Cardiovascular Interventions* 11 (2): 181–191.

Chen, Z.M., Pan, H.C., Chen, Y.P. et al. (2005). Early intravenous then oral metoprolol in 45,852 patients with acute myocardial infarction: randomised placebo-controlled trial. *Lancet* 366 (9497): 1622–1632.

Damman, P., Hirsch, A., Windhausen, F. et al. (2010). 5-year clinical outcomes in the ICTUS (Invasive versus Conservative Treatment in Unstable coronary Syndromes) trial: a randomized comparison of an early invasive versus selective invasive management in patients with non-ST-segment elevation acute coronary syndromes. *Journal of the American College of Cardiology* 55 (9): 858–864.

Eagle, K.A., Lim, M.J., Dabbous, O.H. et al. (2004). A validated prediction model for all forms of acute coronary syndrome: estimating the risk of 6-month postdischarge death in an international registry. *Journal of the American Medical Association* 291 (22): 2727–2733.

Fox, K.A., Poole-Wilson, P.A., Henderson, R.A. et al. (2002). Interventional versus conservative treatment for patients with unstable angina or non-ST-elevation myocardial infarction: the British Heart Foundation RITA 3 randomised trial. *Lancet* 360 (9335): 743–751.

Giannitsis, E., Steen, H., Kurz, K. et al. (2008). Cardiac magnetic resonance imaging study for quantification of infarct size comparing directly serial versus single time-point measurements of cardiac troponin T. *Journal of the American College of Cardiology* 51 (3): 307–314.

GISSI-3 Group (1994). Effects of lisinopril and transdermal glyceryl trinitrate singly and together on 6-week mortality and ventricular function after acute myocardial infarction. *Lancet* 343 (8906): 1115–1122.

Granger, C.B., Goldberg, R.J., Dabbous, O. et al. (2003). Predictors of hospital mortality in the global registry of acute coronary events. *Archives of Internal Medicine* 163 (19): 2345–2353.

Keller, T., Zeller, T., Ojeda, F. et al. (2011). Serial changes in highly sensitive troponin I assay and early diagnosis of myocardial infarction. *Journal of the American Medical Association* 306 (24): 2684–2693.

Lee, C.R., Sriramoju, V.B., Cervantes, A. et al. (2018). Clinical outcomes and sustainability of using CYP2C19 genotype-guided antiplatelet therapy after percutaneous coronary intervention. *Circulation: Genomic and Precision Medicine* 11 (4): e002069.

Levine, G.N., Bates, E.R., Bittl, J.A. et al. (2016). 2016 ACC/AHA guideline focused update on duration of dual antiplatelet therapy in patients with coronary artery disease: a report of the American College of Cardiology/American Heart Association Task Force on Clinical Practice Guidelines. *Journal of the American College of Cardiology* 68 (10): 1082–1115.

Libby, P. (2013). Mechanisms of acute coronary syndromes and their implications for therapy. *The New England Journal of Medicine* 368 (21): 2004–2013.

Mehta, S.R., Yusuf, S., Peters, R.J. et al. (2001). Effects of pretreatment with clopidogrel and aspirin followed by long-term therapy in patients undergoing percutaneous coronary intervention: the PCI-CURE study. *Lancet* 358 (9281): 527–533.

Newby, L.K., Jesse, R.L., Babb, J.D. et al. (2012). ACCF 2012 expert consensus document on practical clinical considerations in the interpretation of troponin elevations: a report of the American College of Cardiology Foundation task force on Clinical Expert Consensus Documents. *Journal of the American College of Cardiology* 60 (23): 2427–2463.

Than, M., Cullen, L., Aldous, S. et al. (2012). 2-hour accelerated diagnostic protocol to assess patients with chest pain symptoms using contemporary troponins as the only biomarker: the ADAPT trial. *Journal of the American College of Cardiology* 59 (23): 2091–2098.

Thygesen, K., Alpert, J.S., Jaffe, A.S. et al. (2018). Fourth universal definition of myocardial infarction. *Journal of the American College of Cardiology* 72 (18): 2231–2264.

Wallentin, L., Becker, R.C., Budaj, A. et al. (2009). Ticagrelor versus clopidogrel in patients with acute coronary syndromes. *The New England Journal of Medicine* 361 (11): 1045–1057.

de Winter, R.J., Windhausen, F., Cornel, J.H. et al. (2005). Early invasive versus selectively invasive management for acute coronary syndromes. *The New England Journal of Medicine* 353 (11): 1095–1104.

Wiviott, S.D., Braunwald, E., McCabe, C.H. et al. (2007). Prasugrel versus clopidogrel in patients with acute coronary syndromes. *The New England Journal of Medicine* 357 (20): 2001–2015.

Case 52: A 55-Year-Old Man with Leg Pain

A 55-year old male with a history of hypertension, hyperlipidemia, diabetes mellitus, and coronary artery disease presents to the office with a six-month history of intermittent left thigh and calf pain. He reports that his leg symptoms occur with exertion, improve with rest, and now limit his exercise capacity to 100 yards. He denies any leg pain at rest. His current medications are aspirin 81 mg daily, atorvastatin 80 mg daily, lisinopril 40 mg daily, metformin 1000 mg twice a day, and insulin. He has been smoking two packs of cigarettes per day for 30 years.

His vitals are notable for a blood pressure of 150/70 mmHg and a pulse rate of 70 bpm. His physical examination demonstrates a regular rate and rhythm with no murmurs, rubs, or gallop. His lungs are clear. He has no carotid or abdominal bruits. His extremities are warm with equal bilateral femoral pulses, a diminished left popliteal pulse, and diminished left dorsalis pedis and posterior tibial pulses.

His ankle brachial index (ABI) at rest is 1.25 on the right and 1.45 on the left.

In addition to offering smoking cessation therapy, what is the next best step in his management?
A Observation
B Start pentoxifylline
C Toe-brachial   index   (TBI) measurements
D Referral for surgical revascularization
[The correct answer is C]

The patient presents with claudication of his left lower extremity and warrants an ABI to establish the diagnosis of peripheral artery disease (PAD). An ABI between 1.00 and 1.40 is normal, between 0.91 and 0.99 is borderline, less than 0.91 is abnormal, and greater than 1.40 indicates noncompressible vessels (a common finding in patients with diabetes mellitus and/or chronic kidney disease). His ABI is normal on the right and indicative of noncompressible vessels on the left. Patients who have suspected PAD and an ABI greater than 1.40 should undergo TBI measurements; a value equal to or less than 0.70 is abnormal and diagnostic of PAD. Pentoxifylline is not an effective therapy for claudication (choice B). Prior to establishing the diagnosis of PAD and identifying the vascular anatomy, surgical revascularization is not indicated (choice D).

The patient undergoes TBI measurements which are 0.85 on the right and 0.65 on the left. He is counseled on smoking cessation, prescribed an antihypertensive medication, and referred to a supervised exercise program.

He returns in six months with persistent symptoms. He has quit smoking, his blood pressure is at goal, and he has completed a three-month supervised exercise program. He states that he wants to have improvement of his leg symptoms and quality of life, but he does not want surgery. He is referred for invasive angiography of his left lower extremity (Figure 52.1).

Cardiology Board Review: ECG, Hemodynamic and Angiographic Unknowns, First Edition. Edited by George A. Stouffer.
© 2019 John Wiley & Sons Ltd. Published 2019 by John Wiley & Sons Ltd.

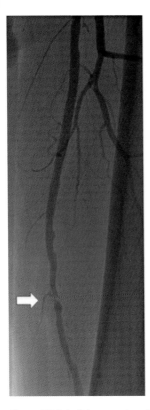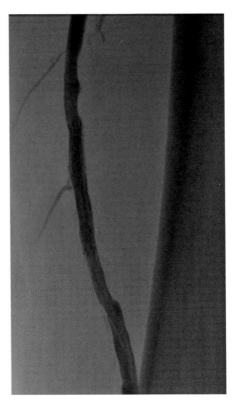

Figure 52.1 Left lower extremity angiograms before and after percutaneous intervention. White arrow denotes site of lesion. Note that the images are at different magnifications.

Angiography shows a severe lesion in the distal portion of the left superficial femoral artery (SFA). What is the next best step in his management?

A Observation

B Referral to a different supervised exercise program

C Endovascular revascularization of his left lower extremity

D Surgical revascularization with a femoropopliteal bypass procedure

[The correct answer is C].

Endovascular revascularization is a reasonable treatment strategy for lifestyle-limiting claudication in the setting of femoropopliteal disease. Observation or a different supervised exercise program may be less effective in this setting (choices A and B). The patient has stated that he does not wish to undergo surgical revascularization for his claudication (choice D).

Peripheral Artery Disease

PAD affects more than 8 million people in the United States and more than 200 million people worldwide (Fowkes et al. 2013; Criqui and Aboyans 2015; Benjamin et al. 2017; Fowkes et al. 2017). It is the third-leading cause of cardiovascular morbidity, following coronary artery disease and cerebrovascular disease (Fowkes et al. 2013; Criqui and Aboyans 2015; Benjamin et al. 2017; Fowkes et al. 2017). Risk factors for PAD include age, coronary artery disease, smoking, diabetes mellitus, hypertension, and dyslipidemia. Given that these are risk factors common to atherosclerotic disease, the majority of patients with PAD have coexisting coronary artery disease and/or cerebrovascular disease (Fowkes et al. 2013, 2017). PAD is associated with an increased risk of mortality, cardiovascular morbidity, and disability (Criqui and Aboyans 2015; Benjamin et al. 2017).

Pathophysiology

PAD occurs as a result of progressive atherosclerosis in the lower extremity arteries and includes a wide spectrum of clinical presentations. Patients can be asymptomatic or have claudication, critical limb ischemia (CLI), or acute limb ischemia (ALI). Patients with claudication have flow-limiting atherosclerotic disease leading to lower extremity pain, discomfort, cramping, or fatigue that consistently occurs with exertion and improves with rest. Patients with CLI have at least a two-week history of lower extremity pain at rest, nonhealing ischemic wounds or ulcers, or ischemic gangrene. ALI occurs as a result of an abrupt decrease in limb perfusion in the setting of acute thrombosis or embolism. Patients with ALI typically have lower extremity pain, pallor, pulselessness, poikilothermia, paresthesias, and paralysis for less than two weeks. ALI can lead to tissue necrosis with subsequent systemic illness and/or death.

The pathophysiology of PAD involves the following potential mechanisms: lower extremity atherosclerosis and arterial obstruction leading to skeletal muscle ischemia and impaired cellular metabolism, mitochondrial dysfunction leading to the production of reactive oxygen species as well as free radicals, and subsequent endothelial dysfunction leading to impaired vasodilation and decreased hyperemia in the setting of increased metabolic demand (Hiatt et al. 2015; McDermott 2015).

Diagnostic Evaluation

History and physical examination are essential in the diagnostic evaluation of patients with PAD. Patients typically have symptoms of claudication, CLI, or ALI but can have atypical presentations with decreased exercise capacity or progressive functional impairment (Hiatt et al. 2015; McDermott 2015). A comprehensive physical exam of the lower extremities includes palpation of bilateral femoral, popliteal, dorsalis pedis, and posterior tibial pulses; auscultation of bilateral femoral arteries for bruits; assessment of the color, temperature, and integrity of the skin; and assessment for wounds, ulcers, and gangrene (Hirsch et al. 2006; Rooke et al. 2011; Gerhard-Herman et al. 2017).

ABI remains the first-line test in the diagnosis of PAD (Hirsch et al. 2006; Rooke et al. 2011; Gerhard-Herman et al. 2017). Patients with suspected PAD should undergo bilateral ABI measurements at rest by measuring systolic blood pressures of bilateral arms (at the level of the brachial arteries) and bilateral ankles (at the level of the dorsalis pedis and posterior tibial arteries) and dividing the higher value of the dorsalis pedis or posterior tibial pressure for each lower extremity by the higher value of the right or left arm. Patients with suspected PAD and an ABI value greater than 1.40 should undergo bilateral TBI measurements. Patients with suspected PAD and normal or borderline ABIs should undergo exercise treadmill ABI testing. In patients diagnosed with PAD, exercise treadmill ABI testing can be used for an objective assessment of functional capacity. In the setting of nonhealing wounds or gangrene, TBI with waveforms, transcutaneous oxygen pressure, or skin perfusion pressure can be used to diagnose CLI. Symptomatic patients in whom revascularization is being considered can undergo duplex ultrasound, computed tomography angiography (CTA), magnetic resonance angiography (MRA), and/or invasive angiography of the lower extremities to define their vascular anatomy and plan for revascularization.

Management

Given that PAD is associated with an increased risk of cardiovascular morbidity and mortality, cardiovascular secondary prevention remains a cornerstone in management. All patients with PAD should be started on medical therapies for cardiovascular secondary prevention and risk reduction. These therapies include antiplatelet therapy, statins, angiotensin-converting enzyme (ACE) inhibitors or angiotensin receptor blockers (ARB), appropriate antihypertensive therapy in the setting of hypertension, appropriate glycemic control in the setting of diabetes mellitus, and smoking cessation counseling and/or pharmacotherapy in the setting of active smoking (Hirsch et al. 2006; Rooke et al. 2011; Bonaca and Creager 2015; Gerhard-Herman et al. 2017).

In addition to cardiovascular secondary prevention, the goals of therapy for patients with PAD are to maximize their exercise capacity, to improve their functional status, and to improve their quality of life. Cilostazol has been shown to improve claudication symptoms and increase walking distance in patients with PAD; on the other hand, pentoxifylline has not been shown to be effective for claudication (Dawson et al. 2000; Bedenis et al. 2014). Exercise therapy has also been shown to improve claudication, increase walking capacity, and improve quality of life in patients with symptomatic PAD (Gardner et al. 2011; McDermott et al. 2013; McDermott et al. 2014; Fakhry et al. 2015; Li et al. 2015; Murphy et al. 2015). Exercise therapy can be prescribed through a supervised exercise program or a structured home- or community-based program. The standard protocol for exercise therapy involves walking at a constant speed, resting when there is mild or moderate claudication, resuming exercise when the pain has ceased, and then repeating these exercise/rest cycles for 45 minutes (Hirsch et al. 2006).

Revascularization can be considered in select patients with PAD based on clinical presentation. Patients with lifestyle-limiting claudication who have an inadequate response to medical and/or exercise therapies or have hemodynamically significant aortoiliac or femoropopliteal disease can undergo endovascular or surgical revascularization for the goal of symptomatic improvement (Gerhard-Herman et al. 2017). Patients with CLI should undergo revascularization for the goal of minimizing tissue loss (Adam et al. 2005; Abu Dabrh et al. 2015; Gerhard-Herman et al. 2017). Patients with ALI should be started on systemic anticoagulation with heparin and assessed for limb viability which is based on motor function, absence of sensory loss, and intact capillary refill (Gerhard-Herman et al. 2017). In patients with ALI who have complete loss of motor function, complete sensory loss, and absent capillary reflex, amputation of the limb should be performed as the ischemia is deemed irreversible and can lead to multiorgan failure and death (Gerhard-Herman et al. 2017). In other patients with ALI, urgent or emergent revascularization using catheter-based thrombolysis with or without thrombectomy or thromboembolectomy is indicated (Ouriel et al. 1994; Comerota et al. 1996; Ouriel et al. 1998; Ansel et al. 2008; Taha et al. 2015; Gerhard-Herman et al. 2017). Following revascularization, patients with PAD should be periodically monitored for assessment of cardiovascular risk factors, lower extremity symptoms, functional status, and hemodynamics with ABI measurements.

References

Abu Dabrh, A.M., Steffen, M.W., Undavalli, C. et al. (2015). The natural history of untreated severe or critical limb ischemia. *Journal of Vascular Surgery* 62 (6): 1642–1651.

Adam, D.J., Beard, J.D., Cleveland, T. et al. (2005). Bypass versus angioplasty in severe ischemia of the leg (BASIL): multicentre, randomised controlled trial. *Lancet* 366 (9501): 1925–1934.

Ansel, G.M., Botti, C.F., and Silver, M.J. (2008). Treatment of acute limb ischemia with a percutaneous mechanical thrombectomy-based endovascular approach: 5-year limb salvage and survival results from a single center series. *Catheterization and Cardiovascular Interventions* 72: 325–330.

Bedenis, R., Stewart, M., Cleanthis, M. et al. (2014). Cilostazol for intermittent claudication. *Cochrane Database System Reviews* CD003748.

Benjamin, E.J., Blaha, M.J., Chiuve, S.E. et al. (2017). Heart disease and stroke statistics – 2017 update: a report from the American Heart Association. *Circulation* 135 (10): e146–e603.

Bonaca, M.P. and Creager, M.A. (2015). Pharmacological treatment and current management of peripehral artery disease. *Circulation Research* 116 (9): 1579–1598.

Comerota, A.J., Weaver, F.A., Hosking, J.D. et al. (1996). Results of a prospective, randomized trial of surgery versus thrombolysis for occluded lower extremity bypass grafts. *American Journal of Surgery* 172: 105–112.

Criqui, M.H. and Aboyans, V. (2015). Epidemiology of peripheral artery disease. *Circulation Research* 116 (9): 1509–1526.

Dawson, D.L., Cutler, B.S., Hiatt, W.R. et al. (2000). A comparison of cilostazol and pentoxifylline for treating intermittent claudication. *The American Journal of Medicine* 109: 523–530.

Fakhry, F., Spronk, S., van der Laan, L. et al. (2015). Endovascular Revascularization and Supervised Exercise for Peripheral Artery Disease and Intermittent Claudication: A Randomized Clinical Trial. *Journal of the American Medical Association* 314 (18): 1936–1944.

Fowkes, F.G., Aboyans, V., Fowkes, F.J. et al. (2017). Peripheral artery disease: epidemiology and global perspectives. *Nature Reviews. Cardiology* 14 (3): 156–170.

Fowkes, F.G., Rudan, D., Rudan, I. et al. (2013). Comparison of global estimates of prevalence and risk factors for peripheral artery disease in 2000 and 2010: a systematic review and analysis. *Lancet* 382 (9901): 1329–1340.

Gardner, A.W., Parker, D.E., Montgomery, P.S. et al. (2011). Efficacy of quantified home-based exercise and supervised exercise in patients with intermittent claudication: a randomized controlled trial. *Circulation* 123 (5): 491–498.

Gerhard-Herman, M.D., Gornik, H.L., Barrett, C. et al. (2017). 2016 AHA/ACC guideline on the management of patients with lower extremity peripheral artery disease: executive summary: a report of the American College of Cardiology/American Heart Association Task Force on Clinical Practice Guidelines. *Journal of the American College of Cardiology* 69 (11): 1465–1508.

Hiatt, W.R., Armstrong, E.J., Larson, C.J. et al. (2015). Pathogenesis of the limb manifestations and exercise limitations in peripheral artery disease. *Circulation Research* 116 (9): 1527–1539.

Hirsch, A.T., Haskal, Z.J., Hertzer, N.R. et al. (2006). ACC/AHA 2005 guidelines for the management of patients with peripheral arterial disease (lower extremity, renal, mesenteric, and abdominal aortic): executive summary a collaborative report from the American Association for Vascular Surgery/Society for Vascular Surgery, Society for Cardiovascular Angiography and Interventions, Society for Vascular Medicine and Biology, Society of Interventional Radiology, and the ACC/AHA Task Force on Practice Guidelines (Writing Committee to Develop Guidelines for the Management of Patients with Peripheral Arterial Disease). *Journal of the American College of Cardiology* 47 (6): 1239–1312.

Li, Y., Li, Z., Chang, G. et al. (2015). Effect of structured home-based exercise on walking ability in patients with peripheral arterial disease: a meta-analysis. *Annals of Vascular Surgery* 29 (3): 597–606.

McDermott, M.M. (2015). Lower extremity manifestations of peripheral artery disease: the pathophysiologic and functional implications of leg ischemia. *Circulation Research* 116 (9): 1540–1550.

McDermott, M.M., Guralnik, J.M., Criqui, M.H. et al. (2014). Home-based walking exercise in peripheral artery disease: 12-month follow-up of the GOALS randomized trial. *Journal of the American Heart Association* 3 (3): e000711.

McDermott, M.M., Liu, K., Guralnik, J.M. et al. (2013). Home-based walking exercise intervention in peripheral artery disease: a randomized clinical trial. *Journal of the American Medical Association* 310 (1): 57–65.

Murphy, T.P., Cutlip, D.E., Regensteiner, J.G. et al. (2015). Supervised exercise, stent revascularization, or medical therapy for claudication due to aortoiliac peripheral artery disease: the CLEVER study. *Journal of the American College of Cardiology* 65 (10): 999–1009.

Ouriel, K., Shortell, C.K., DeWeese, J.A. et al. (1994). A comparison of thrombolytic therapy with operative revascularization in the initial treatment of acute peripheral arterial ischemia. *Journal of Vascular Surgery* 19: 1021–1030.

Ouriel, K., Veith, F.J., and Sasahara, A.A. (1998). A comparison of recombinant urokinase with vascular surgery as initial treatment for acute arterial occlusion of the legs. *The New England Journal of Medicine* 338: 1105–1111.

Rooke, T.W., Hirsch, A.T., Misra, S. et al. (2011). 2011 ACCF/AHA focused update of the guideline for the management of patients with peripheral artery disease (updating the 2005 guideline): a report of the American College of Cardiology Foundation/American Heart Association Task Force on Practice Guidelines. *Journal of the American College of Cardiology* 58 (19): 2020–2045.

Taha, A.G., Byrne, R.M., Avgerinos, E.D. et al. (2015). Comparative effectiveness of endovascular versus surgical revascularization for acute lower extremity ischemia. *Journal of Vascular Surgery* 61: 147–154.

Case 53: An 18-Year-Old High School Student with an Abnormal ECG and a Nervous Parent

An 18-year-old high school student is brought to your office by his mother. He feels well but his mother is worried about his ECG which was obtained during an Emergency Department visit two weeks ago for chest pain. She was told that the ECG was abnormal but no explanation was given. His chest pain has resolved and he is playing basketball on a daily basis without any symptoms.

His vitals are notable for a blood pressure of 124/78 mmHg, a pulse of 68 bpm, a respiratory rate of 12, and an oxygen saturation of 100% on room air. His cardiovascular examination is normal with a regular rate and rhythm, no murmurs, no rub, and no gallop. His lungs are clear on auscultation. He has no evidence of jugular venous distension. His extremities are warm with palpable pulses and no edema.

ECG on presentation is shown below (Figure 53.1). What is your next step?

Right Bundle Branch Block

The ECG shows a right bundle branch block (RBBB) as indicated by a QRS duration greater than 120 milliseconds, Rsr′, rsR′, or rSR′ in leads V1 and/or V2, and an S wave of

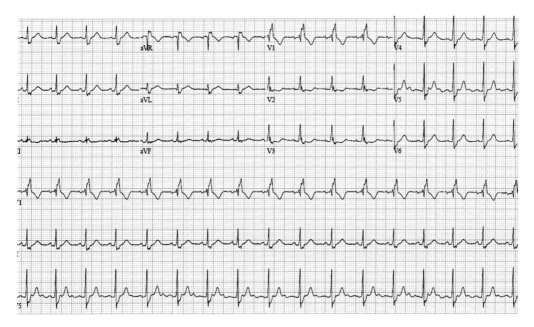

Figure 53.1 ECG from the Emergency Department.

Cardiology Board Review: ECG, Hemodynamic and Angiographic Unknowns, First Edition. Edited by George A. Stouffer.
© 2019 John Wiley & Sons Ltd. Published 2019 by John Wiley & Sons Ltd.

greater duration than R wave or greater than 40 milliseconds in leads I and V6. T wave inversions and ST segment depression are normal in leads V1–V3 in the presence of a RBBB and are not indicative of cardiac pathology. A RBBB in an 18-year-old is not necessarily pathological. In the presence of a normal physical examination and an active teenage (he plays basketball), nothing further is indicated except reassurance.

The 12-lead ECG can provide important clues to the presence of undiagnosed, hemodynamically significant cardiovascular disease in young adults. But the ECG has several limitations – it is neither sensitive nor specific and is rarely diagnostic of a specific condition. It is however readily available and when properly interpreted can prompt further evaluation (e.g. echocardiography) that will provide specific information as to the presence of congenital heart disease or valvular heart disease.

ECG patterns suggestive of hemodynamically important congenital or valvular heart disease reflect abnormalities of one of the cardiac chambers (Bussink et al. 2012). Most commonly, these cardiovascular conditions will alter right heart pressures and/or volumes and thus lead to ECG changes reflective of right atrial abnormalities (RAA) or right ventricular hypertrophy (RVH). Less commonly, abnormal hemodynamics will affect the left atrium and/or left ventricle (LV) leading to ECG changes pointing to these chambers. ECG findings that maybe clues to the presence of underlying cardiovascular disease in young adults include:

- Tall R wave in lead V1;
- RBBB;
- Right axis deviation (RAD);
- RVH;
- RAA;
- Left ventricular hypertrophy (LVH);
- Left atrial abnormality.

When interpreting an ECG in a young adult, it is important to remember that "normal" ECG patterns change as we age. The same ECG findings that are normal in an eight-year-old may suggest congenital heart disease if present in a 28-year-old.

Also, ECG patterns suggestive of cardiovascular disease may be present in well-conditioned athletes but do not necessarily reflect underlying pathology. Incomplete RBBB is common in athletes (14–31% of young athletes in some studies) and is more common in endurance sports (e.g. rowing or long-distance running) or sports with high peak level of activity (e.g. basketball or football). (Kim et al. 2011).

RBBB can be a marker of dilation of the RV (right ventricle) and thus may reflect cardiovascular disease leading to RV volume or pressure overload. The prevalence of RBBB increases with age and it is unusual in young adults. In a study of 237 000 airmen under the age of 30 years, the incidence of RBBB was only 0.2% (Rotman and Triebwasser 1975). In the presence of RBBB, the predominant ST-T vector is usually discordant in the right precordial leads and upright in the left precordial leads and in leads I and aVL. Variations in this pattern may be another signal of underlying cardiovascular disease.

The right bundle branch originates from the bundle of His, courses through the ventricular septum to the apex, and then proceeds to the RV free wall. RBBB reflects a delay in RV depolarisation (via the right bundle branch), usually resulting in a large terminal R' wave in V1 (rSR') and a broad terminal S wave in leads T, aVL, and V6. The World Health Organization (WHO)/International Society and Federation for Cardiology Task Force criteria for the diagnosis of RBBB include: QRS duration >120 ms; an rsr' pattern in leads V1 and V2; S wave longer than 40 ms in V6 and I; normal R peak time in leads V5 and V6 but ≥50 ms in V1 (Marek et al. 2011). The term incomplete RBBB is used to describe the ECG when changes such as those described are present but the QRS interval is between 80 and 110 ms. Note that the QRS axis is unaffected by RBBB and thus axis deviation (either right or left) should prompt consideration of conditions that result in axis deviation.

References

Bussink, B.E., Holst, A.G., Jespersen, L. et al. (2012). Right bundle branch block: prevalence, risk factors, and outcome in the general population: results from the Copenhagen City Heart Study. *European Heart Journal* 34 (2): 138–146.

Kim, J.H., Noseworthy, P.A., McCarty, D. et al. (2011). Significance of electrocardiographic right bundle branch block in trained athletes. *The American Journal of Cardiology* 107 (7): 1083–1089.

Marek, J., Bufalino, V., Davis, J. et al. (2011). Feasibility and findings of large-scale electrocardiographic screening in young adults: data from 32,561 subjects. *Heart Rhythm* 8 (10): 1555–1559.

Rotman, M. and Triebwasser, J.H. (1975). A clinical and follow-up study of right and left bundle branch block. *Circulation* 51: 477–484.

Case 54: Could This Cardiac Arrest Have Been Prevented?

A 24-year-old data analyst without any past medical history collapsed suddenly while in a meeting. He received CPR (cardiopulmonary resuscitation) from his coworkers and was successfully defibrillated. He was taken to a local Emergency Department and underwent therapeutic hypothermia. He was transferred to your hospital for further evaluation and treatment.

Nine months prior to the event, he had undergone a routine pre-employment physical examination and the following ECG was

obtained (Figure 54.1). Could the cardiac arrest have been prevented?

Discussion

Sudden cardiac death is a catastrophic occurrence, especially when it occurs in an apparently healthy young adult. It is thus essential to recognize ECG patterns of congenital cardiovascular diseases that put a patient at an increased risk of ventricular arrhythmias and

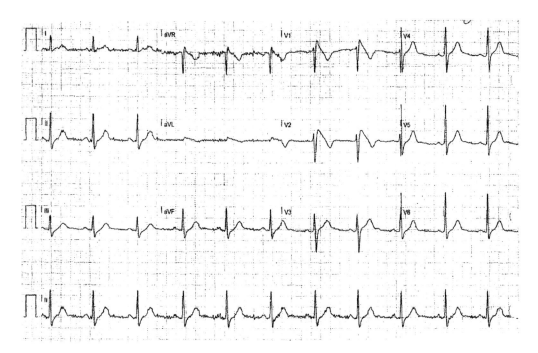

Figure 54.1 ECG in the Emergency Department.

Cardiology Board Review: ECG, Hemodynamic and Angiographic Unknowns, First Edition. Edited by George A. Stouffer.
© 2019 John Wiley & Sons Ltd. Published 2019 by John Wiley & Sons Ltd.

sudden cardiac death. In some cases there are specific treatments, either pharmacological or implantable cardioverter defibrillators, which reduce the risk of sudden death.

There are some conditions that predispose an individual to an increased risk of sudden cardiac death and have a characteristic ECG pattern. Patients with these disorders may be symptomatic or asymptomatic, and in many cases the disorder is diagnosed by an astute clinician on an ECG obtained for an unrelated reason. These diseases can be classified as purely electrical heart diseases (e.g. Long QT Syndrome (LQTS), Wolff–Parkinson–White (WPW), or Brugada Syndrome) or disorders that have an effect on cardiac structure and function (e.g. hypertrophic cardiomyopathy [HCM] or arrhythmogenic right ventricular dysplasia [ARVD]). This discussion is not comprehensive and there are other congenital heart defects, especially those with hemodynamic effects on the heart, which can increase the risk of sudden cardiac death. There are also several causes of sudden cardiac death in young adults that maybe electrically silent. Examples of these disorders include coronary artery disease, coronary artery anomalies, and dilated cardiomyopathies.

This ECG has the hallmark of Brugada Syndrome with a characteristic ST elevation in leads V1 and V2. The Brugada Syndrome is a heterogeneous genetic disease characterized by abnormal electrophysiologic activity in the right ventricular epicardium. Approximately one-fourth of cases are caused by loss of function mutations in the cardiac sodium channel SCN5A (abnormalities in this gene have also been linked to LQTS3). The characteristic ECG pattern of the Brugada Syndrome is ST elevation (≥ 2 mm at the J point) in the right precordial leads. In some patients, complete or incomplete right bundle branch block is present. In others, high take-off ST segment elevation (accentuated J point elevation) in the right precordial leads mimics the pattern of right bundle branch block, but wide S waves in

leads I, aVL, V_5, and V_6, typically seen in right bundle branch block, are absent.

There are three subtypes of Brugada Syndrome. In type 1 the ST segment is continuously downsloping from the top of the R' wave, is not elevated above baseline at the terminal portion, and ends with an inverted T wave. Types 2 and 3 have a "saddle-back" ST-T wave configuration in which the ST segment descends toward the baseline with upward concavity and then rises again to an upright or biphasic T wave (the difference between types 2 and 3 is related to the elevation of the terminal portion of the ST segment). The Brugada pattern on ECG can be either persistent or inducible and the ECG changes can be dynamic, with the same patient manifesting all three types at various points in time.

Diagnosis of Brugada Syndrome depends on both characteristic ECG findings (either spontaneous or inducible) and appropriate clinical findings (unexplained syncope, self-terminating polymorphic ventricular tachycardia, documented ventricular fibrillation, family history of sudden cardiac death at less than 45 years of age, Brugada ECG pattern in a family member, and/or inducibility of ventricular tachycardia by electrophysiologic study). A patient who presents with the Brugada ECG criteria but without the clinical characteristics is said to have the Brugada pattern but not the syndrome. The Brugada ECG pattern is seen much more frequently in men than in women, and there may be an increased frequency in Asians. The criteria that establish a definitive diagnosis of Brugada Syndrome remain under debate.

Arrhythmias and sudden death in the Brugada Syndrome generally occur during sleep or at rest and are commonly associated with bradycardia. Specific factors that have been reported to trigger fatal arrhythmias include fever, antiarrhythmic drugs, β-blockers, tricyclic antidepressants, alcohol, cocaine, and electrolyte imbalances such as hypokalemia, hyperkalemia, and hypercalcemia. Exercise has not been linked to sudden cardiac death. Patients with Brugada Syndrome tend to present later in life than some other forms of inherited arrhythmias (mean age at death = 45 years).

Long QT Syndrome

The QT interval measures the time needed for ventricular depolarization and repolarization but in the presence of a normal QRS duration, long QT intervals occur when there is a prolongation of repolarization. A prolonged QT interval can be either acquired or genetic. Causes of acquired prolonged QT intervals include severe hypothermia, hypokalemia, severe hypocalcemia, hypothyroidism, antiarrhythmic drugs in class 2A and 3, other medications (e.g. antibiotics, antidepressants, haloperidol, etc), severe bradycardia, atrioventricular (AV) block, myocardial ischemia, and neurogenic causes (including organophosphorus). Previously unrecognized LQTS is present in 5–20% of patients with drug-induced torsades de pointes.

LQTS is a genetic disorder that is associated with polymorphous ventricular tachycardia (torsades de pointes) causing syncope and sudden cardiac death. LQTS is a disease of cardiac ion channels with clinical manifestations being linked to over 300 mutations in 10 different genes, with mutations in three genes comprising the vast majority of cases. LQTS1 and LQTS2 are caused by mutations in genes that cause a decrease in repolarizing K potassium ion channels, whereas LQTS3 is caused by mutations of the SCN5A sodium channel gene (Table 54.1). Increased sympathetic stimulation can provoke arrhythmias in LQTS1 and LQTS2 patients. In LQTS1, exercise (especially swimming) and emotional stress can precipitate syncope and sudden cardiac death. Arrhythmic events in LQTS2 can occur at stress or rest; triggering by unexpected loud noises (e.g. alarm clock) is very suggestive of LQTS2. LQTS1 and LQTS2 account for the majority of all LQTS cases. LQTS3 accounts for <10% of all LQTS cases and individuals with LQTS3 tend to experience cardiac events while sleeping. LQTS3 can also be associated with bradycardia and syncopal events can be precipitated by slow heart rates in addition to rapid ventricular arrhythmias.

Short QT Syndrome and Catcholaminergic Polymorphic Ventricular Tachycardia

Brugada Syndrome and Long QT Syndrome are examples of channelopathies, disorders of ion channels. There are two other channelopathies associated with an increased risk of sudden cardiac death which deserve mention. The short QT syndrome is a recently described entity that is characterized on the 12-lead ECG by a QTc of less than 300 milliseconds (ranging from 220 to 300 ms) and the lack of a clear ST segment, with the T wave originating immediately after the S wave. In approximately one half of patients, tall peaked symmetrical T waves are apparent in the right precordial leads. The disorder is familial and a genetically heterogeneous disease. At least six different genes encoding cardiac ion channels and been identified. There are limited data regarding triggers for sudden cardiac death.

Catecholaminergic polymorphic ventricular tachycardia (CPVT) is characterized by bidirectional or polymorphic ventricular tachycardia occurring during sympathetic stimulation. These patients usually present with syncope or sudden cardiac death during exercise or emotional stress and do not have any evidence of structural heart disease. The 12-lead ECG in the absence of ventricular tachycardia is usually normal, although lower-than-normal resting heart rate and a high incidence of prominent U waves have been reported by some authors. Mutations in the gene encoding the sarcoplasmic reticulum ryanodine receptor (RYR2) cause roughly one half of cases, with mutations in CASQ2 being found in a few individuals.

Table 54.1 Conditions that predispose an individual to sudden cardiac death and have a characteristic ECG pattern.

Disorder	Characteristic ECG finding	Gene(s) linked to the disease	Common triggers of syncope or SCD	Miscellaneous
Brugada	ST elevation (≥2 mm at the J point) in the right precordial leads +/− complete or incomplete right bundle branch block	SCN5A in 25%	Rest or sleep, commonly with bradycardia. Other reported triggers include fever, antiarrhythmic drugs, β-blockers, tricyclic antidepressants, alcohol, cocaine, and electrolyte imbalances.	Men > women
LQTS1	Long QT interval	KCNQ1	Exercise (e.g. swimming) or emotional stress	Most common form of LQTS
LQTS2	Long QT interval	KCNH2	Can occur at stress or rest. Triggering by loud noises is very suggestive of LQTS2.	Risk increases during post-partum period
LQTS3	Long QT interval	SCN5A	Rest or sleep	Disorder is also associated with bradycardia
Short QT Syndrome	Short QT interval	KCNH2, KCNQ1, and KCNJ2		Recently identified and thus data are limited; associated with atrial fibrillation
Catecholaminergic Polymorphic Ventricular Tachycardia	Usually normal; lower-than-normal resting heart rate and a high incidence of prominent U waves have been reported by some authors	RYR2 and CASQ2	Exercise or emotional stress	Generally found in children

Condition	ECG features	Genes	Trigger	Notes
Arrhythmogenic RV dysplasia	a) Epsilon waves; b) T wave inversion in leads V1 – V3 in the absence of RBBB; and c) PVCs that originates from the right ventricle	Desmoplakin, plakoglobin and ryanodine receptor genes.	Exercise or emotional stress	Epsilon waves are indicative of localized QRS prolongation (> 110 ms) in V1–V3 and are present if the terminal potential in leads V1–V3 causes QRS duration to exceed the QRS duration in lead V6 by more than 25 milliseconds.
Hypertrophic cardiomyopathy (HCM)	Left ventricular hypertrophy (LVH), repolarization abnormalities (e.g. "strain pattern" in V4–V6), left atrial abnormality, and Q waves in inferior and lateral leads.	Cardiac sarcomere genes (e.g. β-myosin heavy chain, cardiac troponin T, and myosin-binding protein C)	Exercise	
Wolff–Parkinson–White Syndrome	Short PR interval, widening of the QRS complex and delta waves (slurred, slowly rising onset of QRS).	PRKAG2	Exercise	Atrial fibrillation can precipitate sudden cardiac death

Arrhythmogenic Right Ventricular Dysplasia

ARVD is a disorder in which there is patchy replacement of the normal myocardium by fatty and/or fibrofatty tissue. The disease is genetically heterogeneous with mutations having been identified in the genes for desmoplakin, plakoglobin, and the ryanodine receptor gene. ARVD is characterized clinically by ventricular arrhythmias (originating from the RV) and more rarely by RV pump failure. The disease is progressive and as the myocardium is replaced by fatty or fibrofatty tissue the RV becomes dilated and dysfunctional. Arrhythmias and sudden cardiac death are more common during exercise.

Common ECG findings include T wave inversion in leads V1–V3 and PVCs that originates from the right ventricle (i.e. with a left bundle branch block [LBBB] pattern). Epsilon waves, small deflections at the terminal end of the QRS complex that are best seen in V1–V3, are a specific but not a sensitive marker of the disease. Epsilon waves are indicative of localized QRS prolongation (>110 ms) in V1–V3 and are present if the terminal potential in leads V1–V3 causes QRS duration to exceed the QRS duration in lead V6 by more than 25 ms.

Electrocardiogram abnormalities are detected in more than 90% of patients with ARVD. The juvenile pattern of T wave inversion in leads V_1–V_3 is a normal variant in children less than 12 years of age, rare in adults >19 years (found in 1–3% of healthy individuals), but present in 87% of patients with ARVD. The differential diagnosis of these ECG findings includes myocarditis, Naxos Disease, sarcoid heart disease, dilated cardiomyopathy, or right ventricular outflow tract (RVOT) tachycardia.

Hypertrophic Cardiomyopathy

HCM is caused by a mutation in one of the gene-encoding proteins of the cardiac sarcomere. At least 10 different genes have been linked to HCM, but three genes predominate: β-myosin heavy chain, cardiac troponin T, and myosin-binding protein C. Familial HCM is an autosomal dominant disease and present in 50% of patients with HCM; spontaneous mutations are suspected for sporadic forms of the disease.

HCM can present at any age. Many patients are asymptomatic throughout life but others will develop dyspnea, angina, palpitations, and syncope. Symptoms primarily result from hemodynamic alterations which include dynamic left ventricular outflow tract (LVOT) obstruction, mitral regurgitation, diastolic dysfunction, and myocardial ischemia. The most feared complication of the disease is sudden cardiac death, primarily due to ventricular arrhythmias.

There is no characteristic ECG pattern that is diagnostic of HCM but the 12-lead ECG is abnormal in 75–95% of HCM patients. The most common ECG findings in HCM are due to left ventricular hypertrophy (LVH) and include increased voltage and repolarization abnormalities. T wave inversion and ST segment depression with upward convexity is commonly seen in V4–V6 (commonly although incorrectly known as a "strain" pattern), while tall T waves and ST segment elevation are present in the right precordial leads. Because many HCM patients have septal hypertrophy, abnormal Q waves are common. These Q waves commonly mimic those of a myocardial infarction. The increased amplitude of electrical forces from depolarization of the hypertrophied septum can cause deep Q waves in the lateral and inferior leads and taller R waves in the right precordial leads. T wave abnormalities are present in most symptomatic HCM patients. Septal hypertrophy causes the T wave to be directed opposite of prominent septal depolarization force, so the T wave will be positive in leads with a deep Q waves. Left atrial abnormality and prolonged QTc interval can also be seen in patients with obstructive HCM. Atrial fibrillation is the most common sustained arrhythmia in HCM but atrial flutter, ventricular ectopy, ventricular tachycardia, and ventricular fibrillation can also occur.

In summary, there is a wide variety of patterns of ECG changes in patients with HCM including LVH, repolarization abnormalities (e.g. T wave inversion and ST segment depression with upward convexity in V4–V6), left atrial abnormality, and Q waves in inferior and lateral leads. The ECG is not diagnostic but rather serves to raise suspicion of HCM.

Wolff–Parkinson–White Syndrome

WPW Syndrome is characterized by "pre-excitation" of the ventricles. This process occurs via an accessory pathway (also known as a bypass tract), a thin filamentous structure that has conductive properties, thus enabling electrical impulses from the atrium to reach the ventricles without passing through the AV node. Accessory pathways, in general, do not have decremental conduction (defined as rate dependent prolongation of conduction time) and thus do not have the normal safety mechanisms of the AV node in controlling ventricular rates. The most common bypass tract is a direct connection between the atria and ventricles and is known as a Kent bundle although numerous other locations of accessory pathways have been reported (e.g. atriofascicular, fasciculoventricular, intranodal, or nodoventricular).

ECG findings of pre-excitation include a short PR interval, widening of the QRS complex (>0.12 seconds) and delta waves (slurred, slowly rising onset of QRS). Less commonly, repolarization abnormalities (e.g. T wave inversions) will also be present. The PR interval, the time required for the atria to depolarize and the wave of depolarisation to arrive at the ventricles, is shortened in pre-excitation syndromes because the accessory pathway permits the impulse to bypass the AV node. A portion of the ventricles (depending on where the accessory pathway inserts) activates first leading to an initial slurring or "delta wave" at the start of the QRS complex. Conduction also occurs via the AV node and thus simultaneous activation of both ventricles can occur via the His-Purkinje system.

Thus the size of the delta wave and the QRS duration is a function of where in the ventricles the accessory pathway inserts and the amount of relative conduction between the accessory pathway and the AV node.

The most frequently encountered arrhythmias in WPW (in order of occurrence) are: (i) orthodromic atrioventricular reentrant tachycardia (AVRT); (ii) atrial fibrillation; and (iii) antidromic AVRT. The AVRT arrhythmias are due to a reentry circuit that involves the AV node and the accessory pathway(s) and are generally triggered by an atrial ectopic beat. Orthodromic AVRT involves antegrade conduction down the AV node (with retrograde conduction via the accessory pathway) and results in a narrow complex tachycardia since the ventricles are activated via the normal conduction system (the delta wave will disappear during this arrhythmia). In can be difficult to definitively diagnose orthodromic AVRT during an episode of narrow complex tachycardia but clues include a rate that is usually between 140 and 250 beats per minute and inverted P waves within the ST segment indicating that atrial depolarization is occurring after ventricular depolarisation. Orthodromic AVRTs account for most tachycardias in WPW Syndrome. Antidromic tachycardias occur when the ventricles are activated via the accessory pathway (i.e. antegrade conduction in the accessory pathway and retrograde conduction in the AV node). This results in a wide complex tachycardia.

For reasons that are not clear atrial fibrillation is more common in WPW Syndrome than in the normal population. In atrial fibrillation, activation of the ventricles is predominantly via the accessory pathway which causes an irregular wide complex tachycardia as observed in this case. Atrial fibrillation can be life-threatening if the accessory pathway has a short anterograde refractory period, allowing rapid conduction of the atrial impulses to the ventricle. This will result in very high ventricular rates with possible deterioration into ventricular fibrillation and sudden death

RV Outflow Tract Tachycardia and Other Causes of Ventricular Tachycardia in the Absence of Structural Heart Disease and with a Normal Resting 12-Lead ECG

There are various disorders characterized by a normal 12-lead ECG and no evidence of structural heart disease that are associated with ventricular arrhythmias. These arrhythmias are generally not fatal and much more commonly present as palpitations or syncope.

RVOT tachycardia is due to cAMP mediated triggered activity, usually presents between the ages of 20 and 40 years old, and generally is precipitated by a specific trigger. Two typical presentations have been described: nonsustained, repetitive, monomorphic ventricular tachycardia and paroxysmal, exercise-induced, sustained ventricular tachycardia. The most common complaint is palpitations that are triggered by caffeine intake, stress, exercise (during or in recovery), or hormonal changes (in women). In more than 80% of cases, the tachycardia originates from the RVOT, leading to a LBBB configuration with an inferior axis. In most of these cases, the tachycardia originates from the muscular tissue just below the pulmonic valve. A tachycardia can also originate from other sites such as within the pulmonary artery or the LVOT.

The diagnosis of RVOT tachycardia is one of exclusion and other causes of ventricular tachycardia must be excluded. Note particularly that ventricular tachycardia in ARVD may have LBBB with an inferior axis, similar to RVOT tachycardia. Prognosis of patients with RVOT tachycardia is excellent and sudden death is rare.

Other causes of ventricular tachycardia in young adults in the absence of structural heart disease and with a normal resting 12-lead ECG include Brugada Syndrome (the characteristic ECG findings maybe dynamic and not present when the ECG is obtained), idiopathic left ventricular tachycardia (ILVT), idiopathic propranolol-sensitive VT (IPVT), and CPVT. Most cases of ILVT are verapamil-sensitive intrafascicular tachycardias with a right bundle branch block (RBBB) and left-axis configuration.

Further Reading

Drezner, J.A., Ackerman, M.J., Cannon, B.C. et al. (2013). Abnormal electrocardiographic findings in athletes: recognising changes suggestive of primary electrical disease. *British Journal of Sports Medicine* 47 (3): 153–167.

Priori, S.G., Wilde, A.A., Horie, M. et al. (2013). HRS/EHRA/APHRS expert consensus statement on the diagnosis and management of patients with inherited primary arrhythmia syndromes: document endorsed by HRS, EHRA, and APHRS in May 2013 and by ACCF, AHA, PACES, and AEPC in June 2013. *Heart Rhythm* 10 (12): 1932–1963.

Case 55: Why Is This Patient Tachycardic?

You are asked to see a 32-year-old female with recently diagnosed systemic lupus who presented to the local Emergency Department (ED) with complaints of chest pain and shortness of breath. On your arrival in the ED, she is very uncomfortable and any movement causes marked dyspnea. Her physical examination is remarkable for a blood pressure of 82/68 mmHg and a heart rate of 132 bpm. Her neck veins are distended and she has distant heart sounds. No murmur is heard. A pulsus paradoxus is measured at 15–18 mmHg. Her ECG is below (Figure 55.1). What is the next step in her evaluation?

Cardiac Tamponade

The presentation and physical examination are consistent with cardiac tamponade. An echocardiogram would be the next step in the diagnostic evaluation.

The primary hemodynamic pathophysiologic process in the development of tamponade is increased pericardial pressure that impairs diastolic filling. Normal pericardial pressure is zero; any increase can have hemodynamic consequences. Elevations in intracardiac diastolic pressures impair systemic and pulmonary venous return leading to venous congestion and reduced cardiac output. As pericardial pressures increase, a variety of compensatory mechanisms are elicited including sympathetic nervous system activation, which leads to tachycardia, increased ejection fraction, peripheral vasoconstriction, and sodium and fluid retention. The pericardium is a relatively noncompliant structure and thus the relationship between pericardial pressure and volume is nonlinear. Pericardial pressure rises exponentially as pericardial fluid volume increases after a certain threshold is reached. Factors that influence the development of hemodynamic

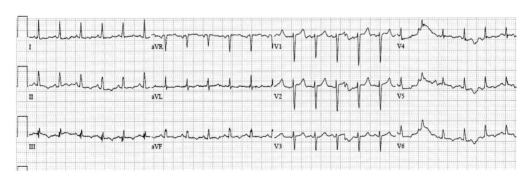

Figure 55.1 ECG on presentation.

Cardiology Board Review: ECG, Hemodynamic and Angiographic Unknowns, First Edition. Edited by George A. Stouffer.
© 2019 John Wiley & Sons Ltd. Published 2019 by John Wiley & Sons Ltd.

compromise in the setting of a pericardial effusion include the rate at which the fluid accumulates, the amount of pericardial fluid, the compliance of the pericardium, the size of the pericardial space, and ventricular compliance.

The hemodynamic effects of increased pericardial pressure occur on a spectrum and cardiac tamponade can be divided into three phases. As the pericardial fluid accumulates, the pericardial pressure rises. Increasing pericardial pressure leads to increasing right atrial (RA) pressure. At this point, clinical signs of tamponade may be absent as the right heart, including right ventricular (RV) stroke volume, but not the left heart, is compromised (phase 1). As pericardial fluid continues to accumulate and pericardial pressure rises even further, pulmonary capillary wedge pressure (PCWP) begins to rise and external compression of both left and right ventricles is present (phase 2). End-diastolic pressures (EDP) throughout the cardiac chambers are elevated and within 5 mmHg of each other including RA, RVEDP, pulmonary artery, PCWP, and left ventricular (LV) EDP. At this stage, classic signs and symptoms of cardiac tamponade are usually seen. In this phase, compensatory tachycardia maintains cardiac output in the presence of diminished stroke volume. Eventually, if pericardial pressures continue to rise and approximate RA and RV diastolic pressures, cardiac output falls and cardiac tamponade progresses to shock with impaired tissue perfusion (phase 3).

It is important to note that increased pericardial pressure occurs on a spectrum and that tamponade is not an all-or-none phenomenon. If elevated pericardial pressures are impairing cardiovascular hemodynamics, the fluid should be removed. The most common treatment of cardiac tamponade is with pericardiocentesis, although rarely surgical evacuation is performed.

Physical Exam Findings

The physical exam can provide clues to cardiac tamponade. Sinus tachycardia and hypotension with narrow pulse pressure are almost always present. Jugular venous distension is usually present with a preserved X descent. In tamponade, venous waves in the neck are not outward pulsations but rather X descents are apparent as a collapse from a high standing pressure level. The Y descent is typically not seen. Pulsus paradoxus is an "exaggerated" drop in systolic blood pressure during normal inspiration (not forced inspiration). Normally systolic blood pressure decreases by 10–12 mmHg with inspiration; a drop in systolic pressure with inspiration >12 mmHg is considered a pulsus paradoxus. This is a common finding in moderate to severe tamponade but is neither specific nor sensitive and may be seen in other conditions including constrictive pericarditis, severe obstructive pulmonary disease, restrictive cardiomyopathy, pulmonary embolus, obesity, and RV infarction.

Beck's Triad is a cluster of findings in cardiac tamponade characterized by hypotension, muffled heart sounds, and jugular venous distension.

Echocardiography in Cardiac Tamponade

The echocardiogram is a useful tool in the diagnosis of cardiac tamponade; however, it is important to note that cardiac tamponade is a clinical diagnosis. The echocardiogram is a relatively quick, noninvasive test, which may aid the clinician to delineate the size, morphology, hemodynamic impact, and location of the effusion. Important findings on echocardiography include:

- The presence of an effusion is the only sensitive sign in tamponade (Figure 55.2). The absolute size of the effusion is not as useful in predicting tamponade with the caveat that larger effusions confer greater risk of tamponade.
- RV diastolic collapse occurring in early diastole is believed to occur only with higher pericardial pressures, however the lack of RV diastolic collapse does not exclude a hemodynamically significant effusion.

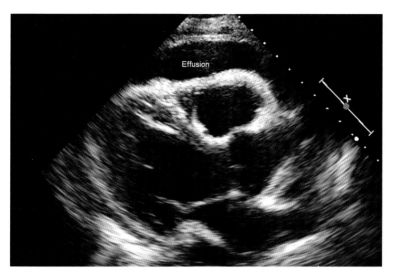

Figure 55.2 Echocardiography in a parasternal long axis showing a large pericardial effusion.

- RA collapse occurring in late diastole or early systole is a relatively early sign of increased pericardial pressure.
- Small chamber sizes.
- Inferior vena cava plethora with attenuated respiratory variation.
- Significant changes in inflow across both mitral and tricuspid valves during inspiration. Doppler transmitral flow velocity paradoxus, a reciprocal respiratory variation in transvalvular right- and left-sided flow velocities, has been thought to be a sensitive sign of tamponade. Normally, there is no substantial variation in early diastolic filling velocities throughout the respiratory cycle. With cardiac tamponade, there are exaggerated increases in right-sided flow velocities and exaggerated decreases in left-sided flow velocities during inspiration A substantial decrease in Doppler transmitral flow velocity with inspiration (>25%) may serve as an indicator of flow velocity paradoxus and tamponade physiology.
- Abnormal septal motion. On inspiration the ventricular septum moves toward the left heart, whereas the septum moves toward the right heart on expiration. The filling of the different ventricles is dependent on the position in the respiratory cycle; an echocardiographic demonstration of pulsus paradoxus.

Further Reading

Kearns, M.J. and Walley, K.R. (2018). Tamponade: hemodynamic and echocardiographic diagnosis. *Chest* 153 (5): 1266–1275.

Mohan, S.B. and Stouffer, G.A. (2017). Cardiac Tamponade. In: Cardiovascular Hemodynamics for the Clinician, 2e (ed. G.A. Stouffer), 234–247. Wiley.

Vakamudi, S., Ho, N., and Cremer, P.C. (2017). Pericardial effusions: causes, diagnosis, and management. *Progress in Cardiovascular Diseases* 59 (4): 380–388.

Case 56: A 31-Year-Old Woman with Palpitations While at Work

You are asked to see a 31-year-old woman who presented to the Emergency Department with complaints of the sudden onset of palpitations and dyspnea. She has no significant past medical history and was feeling well until an hour ago when she noted the onset of symptoms while at work (she works as a paralegal).

On examination, she is pale and dyspneic. Blood pressure is 93/78 mmHg. Examination is unremarkable except for a pulse rate of 150 mmHg. The ECG is below (Figure 56.1).

What is the diagnosis?

AV Nodal Reentrant Tachycardia

This ECG shows a regular, narrow complex tachycardia at a rate of 140 bpm. The differential diagnosis includes: atrioventricular nodal reentrant tachycardia (AVNRT), atrial flutter with 2 : 1 AV block, sinus tachycardia, atrial tachycardia, and atrioventricular reciprocating tachycardia (AVRT; a manifestation of Wolfe–Parkinson–White syndrome or pre-excitation). This patient most likely has AVNRT with retrograde activation of the

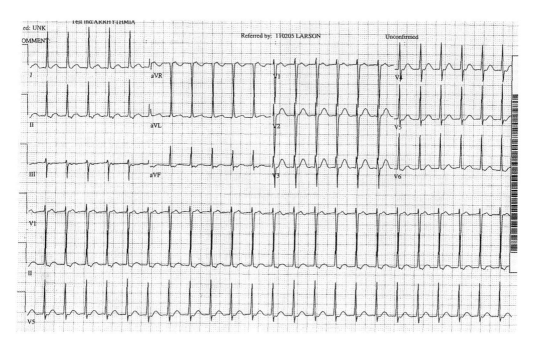

Figure 56.1 ECG in the Emergency Department.

Cardiology Board Review: ECG, Hemodynamic and Angiographic Unknowns, First Edition. Edited by George A. Stouffer.
© 2019 John Wiley & Sons Ltd. Published 2019 by John Wiley & Sons Ltd.

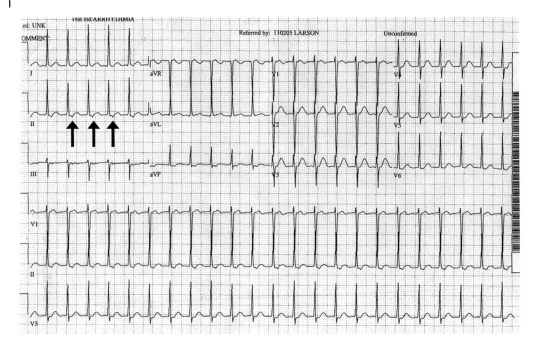

Figure 56.2 ECG showing retrograde P waves.

atria. This is indicated by inverted P waves superimposed on the end of the QRS complex or within the ST segment (arrows in Figure 56.2). In this patient, P waves can also be seen at the end of the QRS in leads II, III, and aVF because they distort terminal vector forces in these leads leading to pseudo-S waves. In some patients, retrograde P waves will cause a pseudo r' in V1 that mimics the RSr' or incomplete RBBB (right bundle branch block).

AVNRT is the most common type of reentrant supraventricular tachycardia (SVT). The AV node can generally be functionally divided into two pathways, with the speed of conduction through these two pathways similar in most individuals. In 10–35% of individuals however, the speed of conduction varies enough between the two pathways that a reentrant circuit can form. The tachycardia is initiated when a premature beat is blocked in one pathway but conducts in the other pathway. Usually, AVNRT is initiated when an atrial premature complex is blocked in the fast pathway and conducts in the slow

pathway, but AVNRT can also be precipitated by premature ventricular complexes. In the majority of patients, during AVNRT, antegrade conduction occurs to the ventricle over the slow (alpha) pathway and retrograde conduction occurs over the fast (beta) pathway. AVNRT is labeled as "atypical" when antegrade conduction occurs in the fast pathway and retrograde conduction in the slow pathway.

Clinically, AVNRT is characterized by sudden onset and abrupt termination. It is more common in females with an increase in incidence between 20 and 40 years old. Episodes may be brief or last for hours and, in the absence of coronary artery disease or structural heart disease, are usually well tolerated. Common symptoms include palpitations, anxiety, lightheadedness, and dyspnea.

In a patient with a regular, narrow complex tachycardia, AVNRT needs to be differentiated from atrial flutter with 2 : 1 AV block, sinus tachycardia, atrial tachycardia, and AVRT. A 12-lead ECG is essential as a rhythm strip provides limited information in regards to P wave morphology. If the P wave is upright in leads II, III, and AVF and precedes the QRS complex, the impulse is most likely originating in the sinus node. In addition to sinus tachycardia, other possibilities include sinus node reentry or sinoatrial reentry. If the P wave is inverted and precedes the QRS complex, consider atrial tachycardia. If the P wave follows the QRS complex, this implies retrograde activation of the atria and thus consider AVNRT, AVRT, and ventricular tachycardia. The P wave can be absent (generally buried in the QRS complex) in AVNRT but this will also occur in junctional tachycardia.

If a patient has a narrow complex tachycardia and is stable in terms of symptoms and blood pressure, adenosine is often given during continuous ECG monitoring. This can serve as a diagnostic aide (flutter waves may become apparent during AV block) and also as a treatment. Because adenosine interrupts the reentry pathway, AVNRT will often convert to sinus rhythm. Patients with recurrent episodes can be educated to use vagal maneuvers (e.g. valsalva, drinking cold water, etc) to terminate episodes. For patients with recurrent episodes who desire definitive treatment, radiofrequency ablation can be curative in 95% of individuals.

Further Reading

Page, R.L., Joglar, J.A., Caldwell, M.A. et al. (2016). 2015 ACC/AHA/HRS guideline for the management of adult patients with supraventricular tachycardia: a report of the American College of Cardiology/American Heart Association Task Force on Clinical Practice Guidelines and the Heart Rhythm Society. *Journal of the American College of Cardiology* 67 (13): e27–e115.

Index

Page locators in **bold** indicate tables. Page locators in *italics* indicate figures. This index uses letter-by-letter alphabetization.

Cardiology Board Review: ECG, Hemodynamic and Angiographic Unknowns, First Edition. Edited by George A. Stouffer.
© 2019 John Wiley & Sons Ltd. Published 2019 by John Wiley & Sons Ltd.